Dignity in Healthcare

A practical approach for nurses and midwives

Edited by

MILIKA RUTH MATITI

PhD MSc BCur (I et A) MCM RGN

Lecturer

University of Nottingham, School of Nursing,
Midwifery and Physiotherapy (Boston Centre), UK

and

LESLEY BAILLIE

PhD MSc BA(Hons) RNT RGN

Reader in Healthcare

Faculty of Health and Social Sciences, University of Bedfordshire, UK

Foreword by

PAULA McGEE

RN RNT PhD MA BA Cert Ed

Professor of Nursing

Birmingham City University, City South Campus, Birmingham, UK

Radcliffe Publishing

London • New York

Radcliffe Publishing Ltd
33–41 Dallington Street
London
EC1V 0BB
United Kingdom

www.radcliffepublishing.com

Electronic catalogue and worldwide online ordering facility.

British Library Cataloguing in Publication Data

A catalogue record for this book is available from the British Library.

ISBN-13: 978 184619 390 3

The paper used for the text pages of this book
is FSC® certified. FSC (The Forest Stewardship
Council®) is an international network to promote
responsible management of the world's forests.

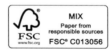

Typeset by Phoenix Photosetting, Chatham, Kent, UK
Printed and bound by TJI Digital, Padstow, Cornwall, UK

Contents

Dedication

This book is dedicated to pre-registration healthcare students and all health-care workers who are committed to promoting dignity in healthcare but have been frustrated due to the lack of a comprehensive text book on the subject that they can use. We also hope that it will be an inspiration to those in training or healthcare workers who have not yet realised the importance of dignity in healthcare.

Tribute to Paul Wainwright

Paul died suddenly on 16 June 2010 as this book was going to press. His very significant contribution to nursing philosophy, ethics and medical humanities was acknowledged in the many tributes from colleagues around the world. Paul will be greatly missed for his generosity of spirit, intellectual rigour and commitment to the value of nurses and nursing. He had the ability to make complex ideas accessible and applicable to everyday practice. Paul was an exemplary teacher, researcher and academic and contributed to the flourishing of many colleagues, practitioners and students. He demonstrated dignity in his everyday and professional lives, offering wise counsel when invited to and giving freely of his time. His contribution to dignity scholarship and research has been substantial, and the field has suffered a tragic loss.

Foreword

Dignity is one of a cluster of interrelated concepts that are difficult to unravel: respect, status, privacy, self-esteem, shame. These concepts form part of the taken-for-granted element of our daily lives. We do not often talk about them overtly, and consequently do not find them easy to explain. When pressed, we tend to draw on negative rather than positive factors. We all know, or think we know, what it means to lose one's dignity by, for instance, being made to look foolish or belittled. Inherent in these feelings is the notion that we have, somehow, been reduced or exposed in ways that affect our self-worth. We are diminished as human beings both in our own eyes and in the estimation of others. Dignity is, therefore, a matter of concern to everyone. It is a global concern in healthcare and fundamental for every patient or client. Quality care requires a commitment to dignity, irrespective of the setting in which that care is delivered.

Certain situations are particularly likely to produce feelings of an assault on our dignity. Our sense of ourselves, the images we project to others, and how we expect them to treat us are easily undermined by sickness and disease. Our bodies or minds no longer behave as we wish and, consequently, we find ourselves depending on others. It is in the shift to dependence that our dignity is first compromised. Pain, illness and suffering threaten our security and lead inexorably to the unmaking of our world (Scarry, 1985).

The behaviour of those to whom we turn for help can make matters worse. Nurses, midwives and other healthcare workers, whose roles bring them into intimate contact with others, can easily undermine their patients' self-worth. Usually this is through sheer thoughtlessness, such as neglecting to make sure that curtains are drawn right around a bed or that someone is not exposed while being transported to the bathroom. At other times it may be due to the pressures placed on practitioners that cause them to appear brusque in their dealings with patients and families. There is no intention in such events to undermine patients' dignity. Nurses and midwives simply overlook the details, turning what should be a caring encounter into an uncaring one.

If these were the only examples, there would perhaps be less need for this book, but, unfortunately, numerous reports have highlighted shortcomings on a much larger scale. Individuals make mistakes and benefit from reminders but where leaders cease to pay attention to direct patient care, systemic failures occur throughout an organisation. Such failure was markedly evident in the inquiry into events at mid-Staffordshire hospitals, where patients were left in soiled sheets, unable to care for themselves. Relatives had to:

> spend extended periods attending to their relatives' hygiene needs. This included having to get the patient to and from the bathroom, washing, and attending to other personal care needs. Little assistance was offered . . . and there was a fear that if families did not attend to such care the staff would not do so (Francis, 2010, p.11).

Patients did not receive sufficient food or drink. Wards were not cleaned properly. There was evidence that patients were treated with 'rudeness or hostility' (Francis, 2010, p.13). The inquiry's report makes disturbing reading. Clearly, something was seriously wrong but it would be incorrect to think that the mid-Staffordshire hospitals are the only example of such failings. As this book makes clear, numerous other reports have demonstrated similar shortcomings over and over again, since Barbara Robb first reported the warehousing of elderly people in the 1960s (Robb, 1967). Time and again promises are made that nothing like this will ever happen again. Time and again promises are broken because human nature does not change; people will not change without conscious effort.

This book is a welcome attempt to address the crux of the matter. Ultimately, the art of helping others lies in the way in which that help is given. This calls for the development of a heightened sense of self-awareness, a process described as *emotional labour* (Smith, 1992). As the term suggests, this is not easy. Working on the self requires honesty and effort in examining our own practice, the humdrum, day-to-day procedures that we scarcely think about but that can so profoundly affect the well-being of others. Urinary catheterisation, administering medication, bed bathing, and forceps delivery may be among the things we do every day, but to our patients they are unusual, often unwelcome, experiences. The attitude and communication skills of the individual practitioner can do much to ensure that these and other similar experiences are not made worse; indeed, I would hope that they are actually improved by careful attention to the patients' dignity (Campinha-Bacote, 2002).

While there have been previous attempts to address dignity, for example through the Dignity in Care campaigns run by the Department of Health and the Royal College of Nursing, there is no other text devoted solely to the subject. This book will, I am certain, make a major contribution to the initial preparation of nurses and midwives. It explores dignity in care from a multi-dimensional perspective. It will promote an understanding of the nature of dignity in healthcare and how dignity can be promoted in practice. I hope that, in years to come, readers of this book will follow the examples of professional leadership demonstrated here by the two authors in compiling this book, and always seek to make the maintenance of patient dignity one of their foremost priorities.

REFERENCES

Campinha-Bacote J (2002) Cultural competence in psychiatric nursing: have you 'asked' the right questions? *Journal of the American Psychiatric Nurses Association* 8:183–7.

Francis R (2010) *Independent Inquiry into Care Provided by Mid-Staffordshire NHS Foundation Trust January 2005–March 2009*, Volume I. Chaired by Robert Francis QC. London: The Stationery Office.

Robb B (1967) *Sans Everything: a case to answer.* London: Nelson.

Scarry E (1988) *The Body in Pain. The Making and Unmaking of the World.* Oxford Paperbacks.

Smith P (1992) *The Emotional Labour of Nursing.* London: Macmillan.

Paula McGee
RN RNT PhD MA BA Cert Ed
Professor of Nursing, Birmingham City University
November 2010

Preface

To our knowledge, no book exists that exhaustively focuses specifically on the subject of dignity in healthcare. This book therefore has two major aims: to explore the importance of dignity for patients and clients in different healthcare settings and to stimulate healthcare workers to understand ways of promoting dignity for patients and clients. This book suggests that healthcare workers should translate dignity into straightforward practical terms and apply these in day-to-day practice. While the book is primarily aimed at nursing and midwifery students, it is also relevant interprofessionally and applicable to those who work in healthcare in general. Thus, where possible, the book explores the concept of dignity in care from multiprofessional perspectives. At the time of writing, the contributors were all based in the UK but they draw on research conducted in a wide range of countries, highlighting the relevance of this topic across the world. Most of the book's content is applicable worldwide although the legislation, health policy and profession-specific content discussed are largely UK derived.

THE CONTRIBUTORS AND THE STRUCTURE AND CONTENT OF THE BOOK

The book's editors and other contributors come from different areas of healthcare, reflecting the importance of dignity in every healthcare specialty. All contributors are committed to the promotion of patient and client dignity and they offer their experiences in research, teaching and clinical practice. Together, they comprehensively address dignity with practical application, drawing on their experiences and knowledge. The contributors recognise that the concept of dignity is relevant to healthcare workers at international level and although they use UK-based scenarios to exemplify their ideas, they hope that readers from other countries will find their discussions applicable to their own settings.

The book has 17 chapters divided into three sections.

Section 1 – Dignity in healthcare: setting the scene

This section explores the meaning of dignity and the context in which dignity is understood and applied in healthcare practice. It would be difficult for healthcare workers to promote patient or client dignity if they did not understand and reflect on the concept of dignity. Promoting dignity is influenced by a number of factors; therefore, it is also essential for healthcare workers to understand how factors such as expectations of professionals, health policy, the care environment and staff behaviours and attitudes affect dignity. This section comprises six chapters. In Chapter 1, Milika Ruth Matiti discusses the importance of dignity in healthcare, reviewing research from patients' and healthcare professionals' perspectives as well as professional guidelines. In Chapter 2, Milika Ruth Matiti and Lesley Baillie explore the concept of dignity and what promoting patient or client dignity entails; they draw on a wide range of literature, including their own research, to explore the concept's varying aspects, perspectives and applications to healthcare. The chapter uses scenarios and reflective exercises to enable readers to relate the content and application of the concept of dignity to their own experiences and healthcare practice. In Chapter 3, Paul Wainwright explores the concept of dignity from the perspective of professional practice and from the expectations of the general public and service users. He explores the popular understanding of the concept of dignity as revealed by the media and everyday usage. He relates this account to the purpose and practice of nursing and examines the implications in terms of the expectations of both professionals and service users.

In Chapter 4, Alistair Hewison commences by explaining how policies are developed, and follows with an examination of England's Dignity in Care campaign, launched by the Department of Health. The chapter explores how 'dignity' has become an important consideration for all who work in UK healthcare. The chapter identifies the dilemmas that occur where policy and practice intersect, and different strands of policy are in conflict. In Chapter 5, Ann Gallagher examines the relationship between care environments and dignity. The chapter discusses the meaning and contribution of the care environment to dignity in care. Two aspects of the care environment are discussed: the physical care environment and other aspects of the organisation, which include the culture and leadership. Some of the concerns relating to undignifying care environments are examined, and examples of good practice discussed. It is concluded that reflection on, and improvements to, the care environment makes a significant contribution to patients, relatives and staff feeling valued and respected.

In Chapter 6, Lesley Baillie explores staff behaviour and attitudes affecting dignity in care, with a particular focus on healthcare workers' communication with patients, their provision of privacy for patients and delivery of fundamental care. With illustrative examples, the chapter reviews research findings of how staff behaviour affects patients' dignity, demonstrating how this behaviour can support dignified care in situations where dignity is under threat. The chapter considers how staff behaviour and attitudes may be influenced by the culture within which they work and how staff can respond when colleagues compromise the dignity of patients and clients.

Section 2 – Dignity in different healthcare settings

This section discusses dignity for people at different stages of their lifespan and when undergoing healthcare in various settings, thus acknowledging that dignity is important to all patients and clients. Readers will be able to select those chapters that are most relevant to their area of healthcare practice, while also developing a broader understanding of dignity across the healthcare spectrum. Each chapter explains the particular factors that influence dignity in this area of practice and illuminates how dignity can be promoted for specific patients and clients.

There are eight chapters in this section. In Chapter 7, Paula Reed explores the meaning of dignity for children, drawing on her ethnographic research undertaken with children and their families in hospital. She points out that dignity for children is often overlooked and that, indeed, sometimes it is considered of lesser value or relevance than the dignity of adults. The chapter explores some of the issues that are pertinent to the dignity of children, illuminating the vulnerability of children, with particular reference to power, control and decision making. The chapter explores the relationship between family-centred care and the dignity of children and examines how the care environment affects dignity, including aspects such as privacy and staff–patient relationships.

In Chapter 8, Barbara Burden focuses on how women's dignity can be affected during pregnancy and childbirth; in particular, she explores the relationship between dignity and privacy. The chapter draws on work undertaken during Barbara's doctoral research in maternity care environments, which used observation and interviews with mothers. She illuminates the strategies that mothers use to deal with affronts to their dignity and what healthcare professionals can do to support them.

In Chapter 9, Wilfred McSherry and Helen Coleman explore dignity with reference to older people and why they are vulnerable to a loss of dignity. The chapter discusses what is important for older people's dignity. This is illustrated with examples of where dignified care for older people might not have been achieved in various settings. The discussion draws on research findings and reports. Practical ways of promoting dignity for older people are provided in the chapter.

In Chapter 10, Davina Porock considers the meaning of dignity at the end of life and the context of death and dying, with particular reference to the UK and current trends of where people die. The purpose of this chapter is to explore why dignity is so important at the end of life and how health professionals can facilitate respect for dignity with the dying person and their family. The chapter is divided into two main sections: the meaning of dignity at the end of life and facilitating dignified dying. The main focus is on dying and death in older age groups because that is predominantly when death occurs in our society. The chapter explores preferences for end-of-life care and examines how healthcare workers can facilitate dignified dying through their interventions, as patients, residents and clients approach the end of life.

In Chapter 11, Candice Pellet examines dignity in care for patients in community settings, taking the UK context as an example. The importance of promoting the dignity of clients and patients in settings such as the patients' own homes, care homes, clinics and general practitioner surgeries is discussed. Challenges faced by health professionals in maintaining dignity within the community are analysed. Community nurses often work with patients and their families over a long period of time, so it is imperative to build trusting relationships in order to promote independence, choice and empowerment on their healthcare journey. The chapter includes case studies relating to community patients with chronic wounds, those undergoing palliative care and those who have long-term conditions.

In Chapter 12, Lesley Baillie explores the vulnerability of patients undergoing acute and critical care, highlighting the patients' anxiety, lack of control and dependency that may result from their acute health problems. She considers the activities and processes that are experienced in acute and critical care and how these can undermine patients' dignity, due to their invasive nature. The chapter considers the challenges and barriers to dignity in acute and critical care, such as rapid patient throughput, workload pressures and technology. She specifically addresses how dignity can be promoted in accident and emergency departments, intensive therapy units, and during peri-operative care.

In Chapter 13, Gemma Stacey and Theodore Stickley focus on dignity in mental health practice, starting with a brief history of mental healthcare. The notion of 'recovery in mental health' is discussed with the promotion of patient dignity in mind. Dignity and self-esteem are recognised as essential to recovery in mental health, although it is conceded that the views of those who use mental health services and routinely feel stripped of dignity are often ignored. The chapter explores the key areas identified within recent policy and research, which require substantial attention if practitioners are to maintain the dignity of people who use mental health services. The impact of practitioners' attitudes towards people who use mental health services in healthcare settings is critically considered, challenging stigma and discrimination.

In Chapter 14, Bob Hallawell examines dignity for people with learning disabilities, focusing on specific aspects of dignity related to the concept of learning disability and the particular context of the promotion of dignity within services designed to meet the needs of people with learning disabilities. The historical and social influences that have created devalued identities for people with learning disabilities and a consequent lack of dignity in their lives are discussed. The author also explores how social policy may both hinder and promote dignity in the lives of people with learning disabilities and he considers contemporary thinking about the promotion of dignity within health and social care settings for people with learning disabilities. The chapter suggests ways that individuals and services may promote dignity through their thinking and actions.

Section 3 – Developing dignity in healthcare

Section 3 is about developing dignity in practice and looking at ways of taking dignity forward. The section has three chapters. The first two chapters focus on the strategies required to assist healthcare professionals to promote dignity in care, through education and practice development, and the final chapter identifies key messages and considers future developments needed, including future research.

In Chapter 15, Liz Cotrel-Gibbons and Milika Ruth Matiti focus on the approaches to education that can be employed to promote dignity in care. The chapter is aimed at both students and educators, with particular reference to pre-registration nurse education, but the content can be applied to other students receiving their initial education in healthcare. In the first section of the chapter the rationale for 'values education' in nursing and the position of dignity within 'values education' are presented, and challenges to dignity education are identified. The educational theories of deep learning, andragogy, constructivism and transformative learning, and their relevance for dignity education, are discussed. It is believed that these theories provide a solid theoretical foundation for the section on the implementation of educational strategies. An example of a programme for dignity education is outlined, accompanied by specific examples of how to implement this programme.

In Chapter 16, Kate Sanders and Jonathan Webster focus on practice development in relation to patient or client dignity. The authors believe that defining dignity is complex and that, similarly, helping practitioners to develop practice in the context of complex work-based cultures and ever-changing services can be challenging. The chapter considers how practice development can enable practitioners to improve dignity in care through creative, transformational ways of learning supported by skilled facilitation. The chapter first provides a history of practice development, to set it into the context of the UK healthcare modernisation agenda. Practice development is then defined and the key characteristics identified. Two pictures from practice are used to illuminate how practice development can facilitate the development of people, practice and workplace. This chapter also acknowledges some of the challenges within complex healthcare contexts and identifies core components that will help sustain and enable ongoing practice development.

In the final chapter, Chapter 17, Lesley Baillie and Milika Ruth Matiti identify key messages from the book, and highlight challenges in promoting dignity in care and areas for development from management and educational perspectives. The chapter reviews research studies focused on dignity, identifying gaps and limitations, and suggests further research needed to underpin dignity in care. The emphasis in this final chapter is on the way forward for promoting dignity in care.

Case studies and reflective exercises

Throughout the book, there are case studies, practice scenarios and reflective exercises that enable readers to explore patient and client dignity from different perspectives. These take into account everyday encounters and challenges faced by healthcare workers. This interactive approach has been adopted to help readers to reflect on practice and consider promoting patient and client dignity in concrete and practical terms, rather than addressing the notion of dignity at purely abstract level. This will allow qualified healthcare professionals and students to explore the dimensions of dignity, enhance their self-awareness and identify practical ways of promoting dignity to apply in their own healthcare practice.

About the editors

Dr Milika Ruth Matiti is a lecturer in the Division of Nursing (Boston Centre) in the University of Nottingham, School of Nursing, Midwifery and Physiotherapy. In 2002 she obtained a PhD with a thesis entitled: *Patient Dignity in Nursing – a phenomenological study*. She has achieved a great deal since completing her PhD but her greatest interest has been in dignity education for pre- and post-registration healthcare students and clinical staff. In 2004–2007, Milika developed and carried out a dignity education programme at a local NHS trust for clinical staff. In 2006 she was part of the Nursing and Midwifery Council working group developing the Essential Skills Clusters (ESCs) for Communication, Care and Compassion. In 2008 she was part of a team developing the Royal College of Nursing Dignity E-learning resource. She has presented and published nationally and internationally about dignity in care.

Dr Lesley Baillie is Reader in Healthcare at the University of Bedfordshire. Lesley's PhD thesis (completed 2007) was *A Case Study of Patient Dignity in an Acute Hospital Setting*. From 2007 to 2009, Lesley was a consultant to the Royal College of Nursing's 'Dignity at the heart of everything we do' campaign, which included an online nursing workforce survey, development of a practice support pack on dignity, and an evaluation of the campaign. In 2010, Lesley was part of a team evaluating the UK's Design Council's 'Design for Dignity' project, which focused on enhancing the care environment through design innovation. Lesley has published and presented widely on patient dignity and is very interested in dignity in different care settings and the education of healthcare students about dignity in care.

Contributors

Barbara Burden RN RM ADM PGCEA MSc Social Research PhD
Barbara Burden is Head of Community Services and Lead Midwife for Education at the University of Bedfordshire. She has a background in midwifery and women's health. She has undertaken research into midwifery supervision and management, provision of maternity care at NHS Direct, and privacy within maternity care settings. She has published a number of chapters in *Mayes Midwifery*, a textbook for midwives, on child protection, preconception care and birth injuries. She has also published on bereavement and the midwife. Barbara is a member of the Royal College of Midwives Research Advisory Group and has worked for them as a research consultant.

Helen Coleman RN Dip Health Management
Helen Coleman is Head of Nursing Practice at Shrewsbury and Telford Hospital NHS Trust. Helen has been a registered nurse since 1979. She has held a variety of senior clinical, management and professional leadership roles. Her field of clinical expertise is in critical care, where the dignity of this vulnerable group of patients is paramount. As Head of Nursing, Helen is committed to improving the patient experience and is currently on the National Patient Experience programme run by the Institute for Innovation and Development. Her project is 'Dignity in Care: making it happen' where her aim is to embed the Dignity in Care challenge into the culture and everyday working methods of her organisation.

Liz Cotrel-Gibbons MMed Sci Clinical Nursing BA(Hons) PGCEA RGN Cert Health Ed
Liz Cotrel-Gibbons is a lecturer based in the Boston Centre of the University of Nottingham, School of Nursing, Midwifery and Physiotherapy. With Milika Ruth Matiti, she was a co-founder of a patient dignity education programme in the United Lincolnshire Trust from 2004 to 2007, which aimed to raise awareness and encourage active involvement of clinical staff in promoting patient dignity. She is involved in facilitating the integration of teaching of dignity in the curriculum for the pre-registration programme.

Ann Gallagher SRN RMN BA(Hons) MA PGCEA PhD

Ann Gallagher is Reader in Nursing Ethics and Director of the International Centre for Nursing Ethics in the Faculty of Health and Medical Sciences, University of Surrey. She was a consultant to the Royal College of Nursing Dignity Campaign ('Dignity: at the heart of everything we do'), and worked with Dr Baillie on the campaign evaluation. Ann's research areas include dignity in care, information giving in mental health, and healthcare ethics. She is editor of the journal *Nursing Ethics.*

Bob Hallawell PhD MBA BA Cert ED RNLD RMN

Bob is currently the Academic Lead for Learning Disabilities in the School of Nursing, Midwifery and Physiotherapy at the University of Nottingham. He began his career in learning disability nursing in 1977 and held a variety of positions within health services around England. He has worked in nurse education since 1987. He has been a member of the Royal College of Nursing learning disability advisory group and an external examiner to a number of UK universities. Bob was formerly Secretary of the Association of Practitioners in Learning Disability (APLD) and is a trustee for a learning disability charity. He is currently a reviewer for the *British Journal of Nursing* and an editorial advisory board member for *Learning Disability Practice.* He has published and spoken at conferences on a variety of topics, including quality in health services, user involvement, curriculum challenges and e-learning.

Alistair Hewison PhD MA BSc RN

Alistair Hewison is a senior lecturer in the School of Health and Population Sciences at the University of Birmingham. His professional background is in nursing, with experience as a staff nurse, charge nurse and nurse manager in the NHS in Birmingham, Oxford and Warwickshire. Having undertaken a number of roles in higher education, including Head of Nursing and Head of School, his current research and teaching activities are centred on the management and organisation of care. His main focus at the moment is a five-year project examining service redesign in three acute NHS trusts. He has written widely on healthcare management and policy issues in papers published in scholarly journals and chapters in edited collections. He recently completed a Nursing Policy Fellowship in the United States and is editor of the *Journal of Nursing Management.*

Wilfred McSherry PhD MPhil BSc(Hons) PGCE(FE) PGCRM RGN NT ILTM

Wilfred was appointed Professor in Dignity of Care for Older People in August 2008. This is a joint appointment between the Faculty of Health, Staffordshire University, and The Shrewsbury and Telford Hospital NHS Trust. He is currently working on a number of projects promoting the dignity of care within the acute healthcare sector. Wilfred has published books and articles address-ing different aspects of nursing care, and has an international reputation for his work on the spiritual dimension. Prior to being appointed to his current role, Wilfred was a Senior Lecturer in Nursing at the University of Hull, where he was also instrumental in creating with colleagues the Centre for Spirituality Studies, of which he was director.

Candice Pellett BSc(Hons) DipHE DN RNA IndNP CPT Queen's Nurse
Candice Pellett is a Case Manager District Nurse at Lincolnshire Community Health Services. In 1999 she obtained a double-award BSc in Community Health Nursing and Specialist Nurse Practitioner (District Nursing). In 2007 she was awarded the Queen's Nurse title, which is recognition of excellence in practice, and innovation and improvement in patient care. Candice works in clinical practice and is also currently seconded to the Department of Health as Clinical Lead for Nursing on the Transforming Community Services Pro-gramme. Candice cares for people with long-term conditions and delivers pal-liative and end-of-life care in the community setting. She is passionate about patient dignity in the community, particularly when caring for people at the end of their lives. She has presented nationally for the Department of Health and has published on end-of-life care.

Davina Porock RN PhD
Davina Porock is Professor and Associate Dean for Research and Scholarship at the State University of New York at Buffalo, where she moved in 2010. She has worked in nursing practice and research in Australia, where she received all her formal nursing education, in the UK, and in the USA, and holds adjunct professorships at Edith Cowan University, Perth, Western Australia and at the University of Missouri, USA. Her focus for research and scholarship is with older people with life-threatening or life-limiting conditions. Specifically, her interest is in understanding the transition from recovery-focused care to pal-liative care and ultimately comfort care at the end of life. Davina continues to collaborate with colleagues at the University of Nottingham where she holds a special professorship and actively participates in a number of nationally funded studies. Davina has published widely on hospice and end-of-life care.

Paula Reed PhD SCPHN (SN) PgDip(Couns) BSc(Hons) RGN
Dr Paula Reed completed her PhD, entitled *The Meaning of Dignity for the Child in Hospital*, in 2007 at the University of Surrey. Paula applied an ethnographic approach to the research based in a hospital ward. Paula remains passionate about the development of a greater awareness and understanding of dignity, especially in relation to children. She has published in peer-reviewed journals and presented her work at national and international conferences.

Paula works for Surrey Community Health, but has followed an unconventional career path. She commenced her working life as a dancer but has worked as a nurse, in acute, community and public health, a lecturer, counsellor and researcher. She is committed to the promotion of health and well-being in children and is currently pursuing play therapy as a way of hearing and understanding the worlds of children in research and therapy.

Kate Sanders MSc BSc(Hons) RHV RGN
Kate Sanders joined the Foundation of Nursing Studies (FoNS) as a Practice Development Facilitator nearly 10 years ago. Prior to this, she worked in a variety of acute and community settings where she became increasingly interested and active in practice development. At FoNS, Kate leads a number of practice development programmes, and has editorial responsibility for the Developing Practice Improving Care Dissemination Series and FoNS website. Kate has actively represented FoNS on a range of national and international events and initiatives. She also works as an external facilitator to support nurses, midwives and health visitors across healthcare practice to develop their knowledge and skills in facilitating and evaluating sustainable improvement and change. She has a keen interest in the characteristics that enable effective development in practice, and in particular the impact of workplace culture.

Gemma Stacey MN RN(Mental Health) PGCHE
Gemma Stacey is a Lecturer in Mental Health and Social Care in the School of Nursing, Midwifery and Physiotherapy at the University of Nottingham. Gemma's research, teaching and clinical practice focus on approaches and interventions that support recovery-orientated mental healthcare. She has published research on the values of mental health nurses and has developed educational approaches that aim to address the factors that challenge the realisation of recovery focus values in practice. These innovative educational approaches have been integrated into interprofessional pre-registration curricula internationally.

Theodore Stickley PhD MA Dip Couns Dip N PGCHE RMN
Theodore Stickley has trained in both counselling and mental health nursing and has worked and taught in both disciplines. He is now Associate Professor of Mental Health in the School of Nursing, Midwifery and Physiotherapy at the University of Nottingham. Theo is a keen gardener, motor cyclist and artist.

Paul Wainwright SRN DipN DANS MSc RNT PhD FEANS
Paul was Professor of Nursing and Associate Dean (Research) in the Faculty of Health and Social Care Sciences, Kingston University and St Georges University of London. He was previously Reader in the Centre for Philosophy and Health

Care at Swansea University. He published books, book chapters and articles on many aspects of philosophy, professional ethics and medical humanities, as well as completing a range of empirical studies. He was a member of two clinical ethics committees and chaired the Faculty Research Ethics Committee and the Royal College of Nursing Ethics Forum Committee. He was also a Fellow of the European Academy of Nursing Science.

Jonathan Webster PhD BA(Hons) MSc DPS(N) RGN

Jonathan is Assistant Director for Quality and Clinical Performance, Bexley Care NHS Trust and Honorary Senior Research Fellow at Christ Church Canterbury University. Jonathan qualified as a Registered General Nurse in 1990 and has worked in both secondary and primary care in the UK and Australia. Up until October 2009 he was a Consultant Nurse, Older People, initially in West Sussex before joining University College London Hospitals in 2005. In this role, he worked with teams and individuals who focused on improving quality of care for older people and their supporters through practice development. During his time there, Jonathan completed his PhD research, which focused upon evaluating a programme of emancipatory practice development centred upon developing person-centred assessment with older people. In his current post he provides the organisational lead for clinical quality within a commissioning primary care trust, along with the clinical lead for nursing. Key to this role is the need to work with stakeholders, ensuring that commissioned services have 'quality' at their core. Jonathan's professional interests lie in developing person-centred ways of working that enable both individuals and teams to work in partnership with service users and their supporters, through practice development and action research.

Acknowledgements

Our idea for this book came about as we identified the need for a comprehensive and practical book about dignity in healthcare. We very much appreciate the positive responses from all the chapter contributors, the high quality of their writing and the wealth of information they have provided for readers. We are sure that all this will make this book informative, enjoyable and stimulating. We also thank all those who have encouraged and supported us, including our families and colleagues, and Radcliffe Publishing for taking our book idea forward to publication.

Abbreviations

A&E	accident and emergency (department)
AMHP	approved mental health practitioner
ANA	American Nurses Association
APLD	Association of Practitioners in Learning Disability
DH	Department of Health
DN	district nurse
FoNS	Foundation of Nursing Studies
GMC	General Medical Council
GP	general practitioner
HAS	Health Advisory Service
HASCAS	Health and Social Care Advisory Service
HCC	Healthcare Commission
ICN	International Council of Nursing
ITU	intensive therapy unit
NDU	nursing development unit
LINk	local involvement network
MP	member of parliament
NHS	National Health Service
NMC	Nursing and Midwifery Council
NPSA	National Patient Safety Agency
NSF	National Service Framework
PDU	practice development unit
RCN	Royal College of Nursing
SCIE	Social Care Institute for Excellence
SCMH	Sainsbury Centre for Mental Health
SWOB	strengths, weaknesses, opportunities, barriers
UK	United Kingdom
UN	United Nations
US/USA	United States of America

SECTION 1
Dignity in healthcare: setting the scene

CHAPTER 1

The importance of dignity in healthcare

Milika Ruth Matiti

INTRODUCTION

The concept of dignity is not new. Many scholars have written on the subject and there seems to be a global consensus that dignity is an important concept to every individual in every society. Dignity is imbedded in Article 1 of the United Nations General Assembly Declaration of 1948, reiterated in 1996 by the United Nations International Bill of Rights, which states that all human beings are born free and equal in dignity and rights (United Nations, 1996). Dignity is reflected in Article 3 of the United Kingdom's (UK) Human Rights Act (1998), which states that 'no one shall be subjected to torture or inhuman or degrading treatment or punishment'; this article applies across society, including healthcare. The 1994 Amsterdam Declaration on the promotion of patients' rights recognises dignity as one of the main rights for patients (World Health Organization [WHO], 1994), regardless of nationality, race, tribe, creed, colour, age, sex, politics, social and educational status, cultural background or the nature of their health problems.

This first chapter highlights the importance of patient and client dignity in healthcare settings, drawing on patients' and healthcare professionals' viewpoints.

DIGNITY IN HEALTHCARE: PATIENTS' AND HEALTHCARE PROFESSIONALS' VIEWS

Worldwide empirical evidence confirms that, for a positive healthcare experience, patients and clients need to feel that their dignity is upheld and that healthcare professionals (most studies are from nurses' perspectives) also view dignity as important for patients and as a valuable part of their professional practice. Confirming the universality of dignity, these studies have been conducted in a range of specialties and some of these are presented next.

Patients in varied hospital settings have identified that dignity is important to them: in maternity care (Lai and Levy, 2002), medical and surgical wards (Matiti, 2002) and for older people in hospital (Jacelon, 2003). Joffe *et al* (2003) surveyed 27 414 patients following their discharge from acute care in the United States of America (USA) to identify how involvement in decisions, confidence and trust in care providers, and treatment with respect and dignity, influenced patients' evaluations of their hospital care. They found that perceptions of respectful, dignified treatment correlated most closely with high satisfaction with the hospital stay, thus indicating that patients who perceive that they are treated with dignity are happier with their overall hospital experience. In the USA, a survey by Beach *et al* (2005) of 6722 adults found that involving patients in decisions and treating them with dignity and respect were associated with positive outcomes. Recently, in Norway, a qualitative study using semi-structured interviews with 12 older people who had had strokes found that being treated with dignity and respect was a core factor contributing to the patients' satisfaction with their rehabilitation (Mangset *et al*, 2008). This main factor was further subdivided into: being treated with humanity, being acknowledged as individuals, having their autonomy respected, having confidence and trust in professionals and dialogue and exchange of information.

In terminal care, a number of research studies have identified dignity as one of the most important issues, from patients', relatives' and/or staff perspectives (Payne *et al*, 1996; Keegan *et al*, 2001; Miettinen *et al*, 2001; Vohra *et al*, 2004; Volker *et al*, 2004; Touhy *et al*, 2005; Aspinal *et al*, 2006). Chochinov *et al*'s (2002a) study of dignity with terminally ill patients indicated that patients viewed loss of dignity very negatively. In a further study, the same authors (Chochinov *et al*, 2002b) indicated a link between loss of dignity and various negative effects, such as psychological and symptom distress, heightened dependency needs and loss of will to live. In critical care settings, nurses stated that facilitating dying with dignity is important in end-of-life care (Kirchhoff *et al*, 2000; Beckstrand *et al*, 2006).

In several other studies, the importance of being treated with dignity has also emerged. Holland *et al* (1997) interviewed 21 patients about their recollections of their stay in the intensive therapy unit (ITU). Participants stated that it was easier to cope with the stress of ITU if nurses treated them with respect and dignity. In a further ITU-based study, Engström and Söderberg (2004) studied the experiences of seven ITU patients' partners, who all stressed that it was important that staff showed respect for the patient's dignity. Clegg (2003) explored perceptions of culturally sensitive care with older South Asian patients who were being cared for in two community hospitals. 'Demonstrating respect' emerged as a core category, with 'Retaining dignity' being a subcategory. The results indicated that promoting dignity was necessary for cultural sensitivity and involved preserving humanity and self-respect in the hospital setting.

Worldwide, healthcare professions have agreed that promoting patient or client dignity is a core element of their practice and this is also evidenced by empirical studies. Kelly's (1991) study aimed to examine what English nursing undergraduates internalised as professional values. The 12 students interviewed perceived two concepts as central to their professional values: 'Respect for patients' and 'Caring about little things'; these both link with patient dignity. Fagermoen (1997) surveyed Norwegian nurses (*n* = 731) with varying experience about their underlying values and found that human dignity was the core value, with all other values either arising from it or being aimed at preserving it. In Yonge and Molzahn's (2002) study, 18 registered nurses from varied settings in Canada gave examples of going to great lengths to preserve patients' dignity in situations in which they were vulnerable, demonstrating the importance these nurses placed on dignity. In Australia, Johnstone *et al* (2004) surveyed 398 nurses regarding ethical concerns encountered in practice. Protecting patients' rights and human dignity was a frequently cited ethical concern, which could indicate high staff awareness of dignity as an ethical issue. Perry (2005) conducted an internet-based study, accessing a self-selected, international sample of nurses (*n* = approximately 200) who were asked to share a story related to career satisfaction. Nurses who were satisfied with their careers believed that they provided quality care; defending patients' dignity was one of the four core values that emerged.

From a professional perspective, international bodies of different professional groups acknowledge that patient and client dignity is important and they have adopted the notion of dignity in their professional charters and policies; here are some examples. The European Region of the World Confederation for Physical Therapy (2003) urges physiotherapists to promote patient dignity at all times in their practice. In terms of midwifery, one of the perinatal principles of the WHO is that care should respect the privacy, dignity and confidentiality of women (Chalmers *et al*, 2001). The International Council of Nurses' Code of Ethics for Nurses (2006) affirms that inherent in nursing is respect for human rights, including cultural rights, the right to die and to choice, and the right to dignity and to be treated with respect. In the UK, under the duties of a doctor registered with the General Medical Council (GMC), doctors are expected to treat patients as individuals and respect their dignity (GMC, 2006). The General Pharmaceutical Council (2010) expects pharmacists to respect the dignity of clients and patients. The Occupational Therapy Association of South Africa (2005) asserts the expectation that occupational therapists should promote patient dignity. These global examples signify that different professions recognise the importance of patient or client dignity.

From these discussions, then, there is a widely shared view among patients and healthcare professionals that dignity is important in healthcare practice. However, while legislation and different professions urge healthcare workers to respect the dignity of patients and clients, the practicalities of promoting dignity for individuals in different situations and diverse settings have not been clearly articulated. There is evidence from different healthcare settings and drawing on patients' and healthcare workers' perspectives that the notion of dignity is neither clearly understood nor appropriately or consistently applied in practice (Porkony, 1989; Street, 2001; Matiti, 2002; Enes, 2003; Jacelon, 2003; Reed *et al*, 2003; Matthews and Callister, 2004; Calnan and Tadd, 2005; Baillie, 2007).

Dignity in care is influenced by multiple and interconnecting influences and, furthermore, the concept is abstract and difficult to define and is consequently not adequately understood, contributing to a lack of clarity about what kind of caring activities preserve dignity in practice (Anderberg *et al*, 2007). Therefore, there is a need to help healthcare workers in practice to identify practical ways of promoting patient and client dignity.

CONCLUSION

This introductory chapter has emphasised the importance of dignity from patients' and professionals' perspectives. The book contributors address the central issues in the current debate on the concept of dignity in healthcare. We hope that the work of the authors in this book will inspire you and help you to further develop your practice as a healthcare worker or student, to better promote the dignity of patients and clients in healthcare practice. We hope this book will be useful to everyone who reads it in their day-to-day practice. At the end of each chapter, authors have provided an extensive reference list which will be very useful for readers to further explore the dignity field.

ACKNOWLEDGEMENTS

I would like to thank Dr Henry Matiti and Professor Jack Mapanje for their valuable comments while writing this chapter.

REFERENCES

Anderberg P, Lepp M, Berglund A, Segesten K (2007) Preserving dignity in caring for older adults: a concept analysis. *Journal of Advanced Nursing* 59(6): 635–43.

Aspinal F, Hughes R, Dunckley M, Addington-Hall J (2006) What is important to measure in the last months and weeks of life? A modified nominal group study. *International Journal of Nursing Studies* 43(4): 393–403.

Baillie L (2007) *A Case Study of Patient Dignity in an Acute Hospital Setting.* Unpublished thesis. London South Bank University.

Beach M, Sugarman J, Johnson RL *et al* (2005) Do patients treated with dignity report higher satisfaction, adherence, and receipt of preventive care? *Annals of Family Medicine* 3(4): 331–8.

Beckstrand RL, Callister LC, Kirchhoff KT (2006) Providing a 'good death': critical care nurses' suggestions for improving end-of-life care. *American Journal of Critical Care* **15**(1): 38–46.

Calnan M, Tadd W (2005) Dignity and older Europeans: methodology. *Quality in Ageing: Policy, Practice and Research* **6**(1): 10–16.

Chalmers B, Mangiaterra V, Porter R (2001) *WHO Principles of Perinatal Care: the essential antenatal, perinatal and postpartum care course.* http://onlinelibrary.wiley.com/doi/10.1046/j.1523-536x.2001.00202.x/pdf (accessed 26 October 2010).

Chochinov HM, Hack T, McClement S, Kristjanson L, Harlos M (2002a) Dignity in the terminally ill: a developing empirical model. *Social Science and Medicine* **54**(3): 433–43.

Chochinov HM, Hack T, Hassard T *et al* (2002b) Dignity in the terminally ill: a cross sectional, cohort study. *Lancet* **360**(9350): 2026–30.

Clegg A (2003) Older South Asian patient and carer perceptions of culturally sensitive care in a community hospital setting. *Journal of Clinical Nursing* **2**(2): 283–90.

Enes SPD (2003) An exploration of dignity in palliative care. *Palliative Medicine* **17**(3): 263–9.

Engström Ä, Söderberg S (2004) The experiences of partners of critically ill persons in an intensive care unit. *Intensive and Critical Care Nursing* **20**(5): 448–58.

European Region of the World Confederation for Physical Therapy (2003) *European Physiotherapy Benchmark Statement.* Barcelona: European Region of the World Confederation for Physical Therapy. www.fysiot.ee/dok/01.pdf (accessed 8 October 2010).

Fagermoen MS (1997) Professional identity: values embedded in meaningful nursing practice. *Journal of Advanced Nursing* **25**(3): 434–41.

General Medical Council (2006) *Good Medical Practice: duties of a doctor.* London: General Medical Council. www.gmc-uk.org/guidance/good_medical_practice/duties_of_a_doctor.asp (accessed 8 October 2010).

General Pharmaceutical Council (2010) *Standards of Conduct, Ethics and Performance.* London: General Pharmaceutical Council. www.pharmacyregulation.org/pdfs/other/gphcstandardsofconductethicsandperflo.pdf (accessed 26 October 2010).

Holland C, Cason CL, Prater LR (1997) Patients' recollections of critical care. *Dimensions of Critical Care Nursing* **16**(3): 132–41.

Human Rights Act (1998) C.42. London: Her Majesty's Stationery Office.

International Council of Nurses (2006) *International Council of Nurses Code of Ethics for Nurses.* Geneva: International Council of Nurses.

Jacelon CS (2003) The dignity of elders in an acute care hospital. *Qualitative Health Research* **13**(4): 543–56.

Joffe S, Manocchia M, Weeks JC, Cleary PD (2003) What do patients value in their hospital care? An empirical perspective on autonomy centred bioethics. *Journal of Medical Ethics* **29**(2): 103–8.

Johnstone MJ, Da Costa C, Turale S (2004) Registered and enrolled nurses/experiences of ethical issues in nursing practice. *Australian Journal of Advanced Nursing* **22**(1): 24–30.

Keegan O, McGee H, Hogan M *et al* (2001) Relatives' views of healthcare in last year of life. *International Journal of Palliative Nursing* **7**(9): 44–56.

Kelly B (1991) The professional values of English nursing graduates. *Journal of Advanced Nursing* **16**(7): 867–72.

Kirchhoff KT, Spuhler V, Walker L *et al* (2000) Intensive care nurses' experiences with end-of-life care. *American Journal of Critical Care* **9**(1): 36–42.

Lai CY, Levy V (2002) Hong Kong Chinese women's experiences of vaginal examinations in labour. *Midwifery* 18(4): 296–303.

Mangset M, Dahl TE, Forde R, Wyller, TB (2008) 'We're just sick people, nothing else': factors contributing to elderly stroke patients' satisfaction with rehabilitation. *Clinical Rehabilitation* 22: 825–35.

Matiti MR (2002) *Patient Dignity in Nursing: phenomenological study*. Unpublished thesis. University of Huddersfield, School of Education and Professional Development.

Matthews R, Callister LC (2004) Childbearing women's perceptions of nursing care that promotes dignity. *Journal of Obstetric, Gynecologic and Neonatal Nursing* 33(4): 498–507.

Miettinen T, Alaviuhkola H, Pietila A (2001) The contribution of 'good' palliative care to quality of life in dying patients: family members' perceptions. *Journal of Family Nursing* 7(3): 261–80.

Occupational Therapy Association of South Africa (2005) *Occupational Therapy Code of Ethics*. Hatfield: Otasa.

Payne SA, Langley-Evans A, Hillier R (1996) Perceptions of a 'good' death: a comparative study of the views of hospice staff and patients. *Palliative Medicine* 10(4): 307–12.

Perry B (2005) Core nursing values brought to life through stories. *Nursing Standard* 20(7): 41–8.

Pokorny ME (1989) *The Effects of Nursing Care on Human Dignity in Critically ill Adults*. Dissertation. University of Virginia.

Reed P, Smith P, Fletcher M, Bradding A (2003) Promoting the dignity of the child in hospital. *Nursing Ethics* 10(1): 67–76.

Street A (2001) Construction of dignity in end-of-life. *Journal of Palliative Care* 17(2): 93–101.

Touhy TA, Brown C, Smith CJ (2005) Spiritual caring: end of life in a nursing home. *Journal of Gerontological Nursing* 31(9): 21–35.

United Nations (1996) *The International Bill of Human Rights*. Fact Sheet No 2. Geneva: United Nations.

Vohra JU, Brazil K, Hanna S, Abelson J (2004) Family perceptions of end-of-life care in long-term facilities. *Journal of Palliative Care* 20(4): 297–302.

Volker DL, Kahn D, Penticuff JH (2004) Patient control and end-of-life care. Part 11: The patient perspective. *Oncology Nurse Forum* 31(5): 954–60.

World Health Organization (1994) *Declaration on the Promotion of Patient's Rights in Europe – Amsterdam*. Copenhagen: WHO Regional Office for Europe.

Yonge O, Molzahn A (2002) Exceptional non-traditional caring practices of nurses. *Scandinavian Journal of Caring Sciences* 16(4): 399–405.

CHAPTER 2

The concept of dignity

Milika Ruth Matiti and Lesley Baillie

INTRODUCTION

To be able to promote dignity in healthcare, we need to understand the meaning of dignity. However, while dignity is frequently referred to in the media and health policy, it is by no means a universally understood concept. The French philosopher Gabriel Marcel believed that the 'mysterious principle at the heart of human dignity' cannot be preserved unless its 'sacred quality' is made precise (Marcel, 1963, p.128). Shotton and Seedhouse (1998) suggested that dignity is a vague and poorly defined concept, warning that unless dignity's meaning is clear, it can disappear beneath more tangible and measurable priorities. The Social Care Institute for Excellence (SCIE; 2006) pointed out that although defining dignity may be difficult, 'people know when they have not been treated with dignity and respect'.

In this chapter we will therefore explore the concept of dignity, drawing on a range of perspectives. We start with reflective exercises to enable you to explore your own understanding of dignity and develop a personal definition of dignity. The chapter continues by reviewing definitions of dignity from the healthcare literature, drawing on concept analyses and research with patients and healthcare workers. We will use scenarios to help you to understand how the concept of dignity is perceived by patients or clients. The chapter also aims to explore factors that influence how people perceive their own dignity.

LEARNING OUTCOMES

By the end of the chapter you will be able to:
➤ recognise your own understanding and perceptions of dignity
➤ discuss how dignity has been defined in the healthcare literature and the core elements of dignity
➤ understand how dignity is maintained and promoted through other related concepts.

REFLECTIONS ON YOUR OWN UNDERSTANDING OF DIGNITY

We suggest that you start by reflecting on your own understanding of dignity by carrying out Reflective activity 2.1. The activity guides you to reflect on what 'dignity' means to you and then to ask a friend to do likewise. You will then have insights into your own understanding of dignity and how understandings of dignity might differ between two individuals.

Reflective activity 2.1 The meaning of dignity

1. Write down some notes on what dignity means to you.
2. Now, read through what you have written and list words that describe dignity for you.
3. Reflect on each of the words in your list:
    a What exactly does each word mean?
    b Did you find it easy or difficult to define what dignity means?
4. How would you need to behave in order to promote dignity as you have described it?
5. How should other people promote the kind of dignity you have in mind? Look again at each word you have listed and state exactly how you would like others to promote it.
6. *Where* did you learn the behaviour that relates to your definition of dignity?
7. *How* did you learn the behaviour that relates to your definition of dignity?
    When you are satisfied that you have fully explored your understanding of dignity, ask a friend to do the same exercises (1–7) and compare your notes.
8. How do your views on the meaning of dignity compare with your friend's?
9. Were there any differences or similarities between you and your friend's views about the behaviour that promotes dignity?
10. Were there any differences or similarities in how and where you and your friend learnt the behaviour relating to dignity?
11. If there are differences in your views, discuss the reasons why with your friend.
12. In your own words, write a summary of what you have learnt from this exercise.

The next sections of this chapter explore published definitions of dignity.

DEFINITIONS OF DIGNITY

There are definitions of dignity in dictionaries, while other definitions have developed from philosophical exploration and concept analyses and through research.

Dictionary definitions of dignity

Collins English Dictionary (2003) states that the word dignity comes from two Latin words: *'dignus'*, meaning worth, and *'dignitas,'* meaning merit. Most definitions of dignity have assumed the relevance of these two roots, as you will see if you look up 'dignity' in a dictionary or thesaurus. Now carry out Reflective activity 2.2.

Reflective activity 2.2 Dictionary and thesaurus definitions of dignity

Look up 'dignity' in a dictionary (hard copy and/or an online dictionary) and a thesaurus and consider:

➤ how do the definitions and words in the dictionary or thesaurus relate to the Latin meanings of 'worth' and 'merit'?
➤ how helpful are the definitions in clarifying what the concept of dignity means?
➤ how applicable are these definitions in relation to dignity in healthcare?

You will probably have found that most words in definitions of dignity in dictionaries, and the words listed in the thesaurus, are abstract and need defining themselves. Some definitions include internal qualities like having pride in oneself, self-respect and self-esteem. Others relate to how one is viewed in society, including notions of nobility and being in an esteemed position. This exercise illustrates that dignity can be defined and interpreted in different ways; some of these may be more applicable to healthcare than others. We will next examine the meaning of dignity proposed in philosophical and theoretical explorations.

Theories of dignity

The German philosopher Immanuel Kant's views on dignity have been widely referred to in discussions of the meaning of dignity. He defined dignity as an intrinsic, unconditional and incomparable worth or worthiness that should not be compared with things that have economic value because, unlike market value, a person's value does not depend upon usefulness and cannot be replaced (Kant, 1948). Kant argued that dignity should be accorded on the basis of ability to reason and that as humans are able to reason, they possess dignity (Kant, 1909). He related rationality with autonomy: 'Autonomy then is the basis of the dignity of human and of every rational nature' (Kant, 1909, p.54). However, Beauchamp (2001) asserted that Kant's (1909) philosophy failed to acknowledge the dignity of those who lack the capacity for autonomy, which is particularly relevant in healthcare. A number of definitions have been influenced by Kant's ideas about dignity however.

Nordenfelt (2003) developed a theoretical framework for dignity from reviewing the literature. His work was related to dignity in older people and is further discussed in Chapter 9. He proposed four categories of dignity:

➤ *Menschenwürde* (a German word) refers to the dignity that each individual has by virtue of being human; everyone has this human value to the same degree regardless of sex, age, race or religion

➤ *dignity as merit* includes rank in society, earned or inherited; this also entails a set of rights and honours installed in this position – for example, a king, queen, chiefs, lawyers – and therefore this varies from one person to the other. This definition closely relates to some of the dictionary definitions found in Reflective activity 2.2

➤ *dignity of moral stature* includes respect of oneself as a moral human being and respect from others related to performances and attitudes, and may vary in relation to one's own acts

➤ *dignity of personal identity* focuses on human beings' self-respect, including notions of integrity and autonomy, and may be violated when a person is prevented from doing what they want to do or are entitled to do, or by physical assault and humiliation.

In a later paper, Nordenfelt and Edgar (2005) emphasised that while *Menschenwürde* (human dignity) cannot be diminished or lost while a person is alive, the presence and degree of the other three types of dignity varies in each individual. They acknowledged that dignity of identity is most relevant in the context of illness, as disability restricts autonomy and threatens personal identity. Baillie (2009) argued that the categories 'dignity as merit' and 'dignity as moral stature' have questionable relevance to healthcare because all patients should be treated with respect for dignity, regardless of perceived merit or moral status. Wainwright and Gallagher have also critiqued Nordenfelt's analysis (*see* Chapter 3 of this book).

Jacobson's (2007) analysis identified two distinct meanings of dignity: human dignity (a value that belongs to every human being because they are human) and social dignity. Jacobson (2007) explained that social dignity is experienced through interaction and, while human dignity cannot be removed, social dignity can be 'lost or gained, threatened, violated, or promoted' (p.295). She elaborated that social dignity always arises in a social context and comprises two linked elements: 'dignity-of-self' (includes self-confidence and self-respect), which is created through interaction, and 'dignity-in-relation', which concerns the conveyance of worth to others and is situated in time and place. Jacobson (2007) also asserted that traditional definitions of dignity relating to status and merit (as in Nordenfelt's model) are included in social dignity; thus, this broad category of social dignity encompasses various interpretations. Jacobson (2007) suggested that being clear about whether human or social dignity is being discussed may help to reduce some of the vagueness associated with dignity. She also asserted that the concept of human dignity can be used to argue for the right to health.

Concept analyses of dignity

Concept analyses of dignity have mostly comprised theoretical analysis and literature reviews (Johnson, 1998; Fenton and Mitchell, 2002; Griffin-Heslin, 2005; Coventry, 2006), but a few included views from convenience samples of students (Mairis, 1994; Jacobs, 2000) or friends, colleagues and family (Haddock, 1996; Marley, 2005). One United States (US)-based concept analysis of dignity in older people appropriately included focus groups with older people (Jacelon *et al*, 2004). Some concept analyses drew on popular literature, visual art and poetry, recognising that the word 'dignity' is used in a broad context. The concept analyses highlight that dignity is complex and multidimensional. Mairis's (1994) concept analysis identified critical attributes of dignity as being the maintenance of self-respect, self-esteem and appreciation of individual standards. Her definition referred to individuals being able to apply control or choice over their own behaviour and surroundings and how others treat them. The definition also included being able to understand information and make decisions and feeling comfortable with oneself, both physically and from a psychosocial perspective.

Haddock (1996) concluded that the dignified self comprises self-respect; self-confidence; self-control; control of environment; pride of self; being trustworthy, happy with self, humorous, autonomous, independent, private; positive self; striving to keep boundary, integrity and identity of self when under attack. Her operational definition of dignity included feeling, and being treated as being, important and valuable when in situations that are considered threatening. The definition also highlighted the link between one's own dignity and the ability to promote the dignity of others; this is an important consideration for healthcare professionals working with patients (*see* Chapter 3).

Fenton and Mitchell's (2002) concept analysis of dignity in older people included, like Mairis's concept analysis, control, choice and decision making. However, they also included being valued as an individual and feeling comfortable (physically, emotionally and spiritually). Jacelon *et al*'s (2004) concept analysis also focused on older people. Their definition included dignity as part of being human, dignity as an attribute of self, and related concepts and 'behavioural dignity' with attributes including self-worth, self-respect and pride. Marley's (2005) concept analysis of dignity led him to emphasise dignity as being two-way: 'a quality that existed both in and for people; that it is both a possession and a gift' (p.84).

In the next section we focus on healthcare research which gained understanding of dignity from patients' and healthcare professionals' perspectives.

Research findings about the meaning of dignity

Researchers have often focused on experiences of dignity rather than the meaning of dignity; here we review studies that have specifically explored what dignity means. Nearly all studies were qualitative, involving in-depth interviews with patients, healthcare professionals (mostly nurses) and occasionally relatives; a few used observation too. Understanding the meaning of dignity in healthcare is clearly of universal concern as researchers have explored the meaning of dignity in the US (Porkony, 1989; Jacelon, 2003), the UK (Seedhouse and Gallagher, 2002; Matiti, 2002; Enes 2003; Reed *et al*, 2003; Baillie, 2009), Sweden (Randers and Mattiasson, 2004), Canada (Chochinov *et al*, 2002) and Europe – the 'Dignity and Older Europeans' project (Ariño-Blasco *et al*, 2005; Bayer *et al*, 2005; Stratton and Tadd, 2005). Most studies were conducted with adult hospital patients but Enes' study was hospice based, Chochinov *et al*'s (2002) research was in a palliative care unit, and Reed *et al*'s (2003) study was with children (*see* Chapter 8). The 'Dignity in Older Europeans' project, based on Nordenfelt's (2003) theoretical framework, included members of the public as well as healthcare professionals. Both chapter authors have conducted their own doctoral research into the meaning of dignity and we present some of these findings here.

Using a phenomenological approach, Matiti (2002) conducted interviews with patients and nurses about dignity in hospital wards in England. Patients described their concept of dignity as: privacy, confidentiality, need for information, choice, involvement in care, independence, forms of address, decency, control, respect and nurse–patient communication. Patients also described dignity as something everyone has, that it is about self-worth and personal standards, how they present themselves and are perceived by others. Privacy was highly rated by all participants as a main attribute of dignity. Matiti (2002) found that patients went through a process of adjustment in hospital, which she referred to as 'perceptual adjustment level' and thus she developed the following definition:

> Patient dignity is the fulfilment of patients' expectations in terms of values within each patient's perceptual adjustment level, taking into account the hospital environment (Matiti, 2002, p.105).

The definition indicates the individuality of dignity to patients, implying that the meaning of dignity varies according to what the patient expects, how they have adjusted to being in hospital, and the impact of the hospital setting on them.

Baillie (2007) conducted a multi-method qualitative case study on a hospital ward in England using participant observation, interviews with nurses and patients and documentary analysis. The central component of dignity in hospital emerged as being how patients feel, which was linked with their physical presentation and behaviour towards and from others. Feelings associated with dignity related to feeling comfortable (for example, safe, happy, relaxed), in control (for example, confident, able to cope) and valued (for example, of consequence, cared about). About half the patients and most staff associated dignity with appearance: patients being dressed appropriately and not having their bodies exposed. Many participants associated dignity with behaviour towards and from others, as this influenced how comfortable patients felt and whether they felt valued. Most patients and staff referred to behaviour, with 'respect' being the most commonly used term. Some felt that dignity entailed reciprocity: mutually respectful behaviour. Some staff and patients identified privacy as a behaviour associated with the meaning of dignity. Baillie's definition of dignity, developed from the patients' expressed meanings of dignity, is:

> Patient dignity is feeling valued and comfortable psychologically with one's physical presentation and behaviour, level of control over the situation, and the behaviour of other people in the environment (Baillie, 2007, p.247).

There are similarities between the findings of our doctoral research and with the concept analyses and other research studies, as we will discuss next.

The meaning of dignity: a summary from the literature

For our review we summarise the key themes as:

➤ *dignity is inherent in human beings* (Matiti, 2002; Nordenfelt, 2003; Jacelon, 2003; Reed *et al*, 2003; Jacelon *et al*, 2004; Griffin-Heslin, 2005; Marley, 2005; Jacobson, 2007)

➤ *dignity is dynamic*: patients adjust their perceptions of dignity during hospitalisation (Matiti, 2002; Jacelon, 2003) and as illness progresses (Enes, 2003)

➤ *dignity is an internal quality*: an aspect of self (Haddock, 1996), self-dignity (Jacelon, 2003), dignity-of-self (Jacobson, 2007), an attribute of the self (Jacelon *et al*, 2004), a possession (Marley, 2005), and closely linked to each patient's individuality, their feelings and uniqueness as an individual (Mairis, 1994; Fenton and Mitchell, 2002; Marley, 2005)

➤ *dignity relates to feelings*: self-esteem (Matiti, 2002; Chochinov *et al*, 2002; Enes, 2003), self-worth (Matiti, 2002; Enes, 2003), pride (Seedhouse and Gallagher, 2002; Chochinov *et al*, 2002; Matiti, 2002), confidence (Seedhouse and Gallagher, 2002; Baillie, 2007), self-respect (Seedhouse and Gallagher, 2002; Chochinov *et al*, 2002; Matiti, 2002; Baillie, 2007), feeling important and valuable (Baillie, 2007), being happy with self (Baillie, 2007), well-being (Chochinov *et al*, 2002; Baillie, 2007), hope (Chochinov *et al*, 2002) and feeling comfortable (Fenton and Mitchell, 2002; Baillie, 2007)

➤ *dignity relates to behaviour*: behavioural dignity (Jacelon *et al*, 2004), dignity-in-relation (Jacobson, 2007), a gift (Marley, 2005). Examples are: behaving according to one's personal standards (Matiti, 2002; Jacelon, 2003; Baillie, 2007), courteousness (Matiti, 2002; Baillie, 2007), conveying respect (Seedhouse and Gallagher, 2002; Matiti, 2002; Enes, 2003; Jacelon, 2003), reciprocal respect (Jacelon *et al*, 2004; Baillie, 2007) and treating people as individuals (Enes, 2003; Baillie, 2007), as competent adults (Seedhouse and Gallagher, 2002) and as important and valuable (Haddock, 1996; Baillie, 2007)

➤ *dignity and relationships*: interpersonal dignity (Jacelon, 2003) and relationships involving reciprocal behaviour (Enes, 2003; Jacelon, 2003; Reed *et al*, 2003; Baillie, 2007)

➤ *control as a component of dignity* (Matiti, 2002; Jacelon, 2003; Reed *et al*, 2003; Baillie, 2007). Related concepts are: autonomy (Chochinov *et al*, 2002; Randers and Mattiasson, 2004) and independence (Pokorny, 1989; Seedhouse and Gallagher, 2002; Chochinov *et al*, 2002; Matiti, 2002; Enes, 2003; Baillie, 2007)

➤ *presentation of self in public*: physical appearance (Seedhouse and Gallagher, 2002; Chochinov *et al*, 2002; Matiti, 2002; Enes, 2003; Baillie, 2007) and modesty (Matiti, 2002; Baillie, 2007)

➤ *privacy* (Porkony, 1989; Seedhouse and Gallagher, 2002; Chochinov *et al*, 2002; Matiti, 2002; Enes, 2003; Reed *et al*, 2003; Jacelon, 2003; Randers and Mattiasson, 2004; Baillie, 2007). Other examples are: being private and able to keep one's boundaries (Haddock, 1996), protecting privacy to convey respect (Jacobs, 2000; Jacelon, 2003; Griffin-Heslin, 2005), being in control of one's own privacy (Marley, 2005).

Following this review, now carry out Reflective activity 2.3.

ATTRIBUTES OF DIGNITY

The previous section indicated that other concepts have been used to describe the concept of dignity and that despite studies being carried out in a wide range of countries, there are some similar ideas about dignity. Chinn and Jacobs (1983) state that if a concept is difficult to define, its meaning can be inferred from other theoretical concepts, which they call 'attributes'. These are concepts that appear repeatedly in the literature to describe a concept. It may therefore

Reflective activity 2.3 Comparing definitions of dignity

Look back at the definitions and meanings of dignity included in this section and list all the common words that are used. Now compare these to the words you used in the definition you developed in Reflective activity 2.1.

➤ Do any of these definitions match with your definitions?
➤ Do the definitions from the literature make the concept of dignity clearer to you?
➤ Has the literature review led to any different perspectives of dignity for you?
➤ What conclusions can you draw?

be easier to describe or define the notion of dignity by using attributes but these attributes are also abstract and need defining further. Attributes associated with dignity include respect, privacy, autonomy and worth but what do they mean exactly? Think critically and look at the list of attributes that you compiled in Reflective activity 2.1 to describe the concept of dignity. Now consider: is it more practical to explain what dignity means by using its attributes?

Owing to the abstract nature of the concept of dignity, you will find that sometimes attributes of dignity (for example, privacy, respect, worth) are used interchangeably with dignity or attached to dignity (see examples in Box 2.1). This interchangeable use of the concept of dignity with its attributes further blurs the meaning of dignity and can cause confusion. In Chapter 3, Paul Wainwright explores this issue further, drawing on a range of literature and media reports.

BOX 2.1 *Examples of how dignity is used interchangeably or linked with its attributes*

1. The rights designated as human are justifiable by reference to the principle that all humans are beings with intrinsic worth and dignity (Blackstone, 1970, pp.34–5)
2. *Privacy and Dignity – A Report by the Chief Nursing Officer into Mixed Sex Accommodation in Hospitals* (Department of Health, 2007)
3. Privacy and dignity of cancer patients: a qualitative study of patients' privacy in UK National Health Service patient care settings (Woogara, 2005)
4. Care of the body: maintaining dignity and respect (Bernick *et al*, 2002)

At this juncture, you are probably realising that it is through its attributes that dignity is maintained and so it is important to discuss what influences perceptions of these attributes in relation to one's dignity. A person's background, their age, previous experience and social standing in the community might influence their perception of dignity. The situation in which a person finds himself or herself also influences the way they perceive the maintenance of their dignity. Another factor is hospitalisation, as the type of illness and treatment also influences a person's perception of their dignity. Now consider the scenario and questions in Reflective activity 2.4 , which will help you to explore how a patient might perceive their dignity and what might influence their perception.

Reflective activity 2.4 Perceptions of dignity

Mrs Smith, an 80-year-old widow who had worked as a nurse and rose through the ranks to retire as a matron, has been admitted, with a bladder tumour, onto a ward she had worked on 40 years before. She is having difficulties controlling her bladder and cannot go to the toilet unassisted as she has arthritis, which limits her mobility. She is told that she needs a urinary catheter. A young nurse goes over to her and calls her by her first name. You overhear her talking to the patient in the next bed: 'Things have changed these days, during my time patients were addressed properly using their surnames. I personally do not feel respected being addressed by my first name; at least I should be asked if I mind. This is how I have been brought up'.

➤ First, identify some attributes through which Mrs Smith's dignity might be promoted.
➤ Can you identify what would influence her perception regarding the maintenance of her dignity while in hospital?

The factors influencing dignity will be discussed further in the next section.

FACTORS INFLUENCING PERCEPTIONS OF THE ATTRIBUTES OF DIGNITY

Each community or family has its own perception and sets its own standards regarding attributes of dignity, such as respect, privacy and forms of address. Take, for example, the attribute 'respect'. Most families teach their children the expected mode of behaviour that constitutes respect; that is, how to respect oneself and others. Other factors that influence a child's perception and understanding of respect include institutions such as schools. As we grow up, the environment in which we live, including the people we work, live and socialise with, continues to influence our understanding of the concept of respect. Healthcare professionals' understanding of dignity is influenced by their education and experience of working with patients in healthcare settings.

Regarding the attribute of privacy or 'being decent': children are taught dress codes, which in some cultures require covering almost the whole body. As they grow up, children learn these shared standards of beliefs and values which are internalised and become part of a person's self-concept. Self-concept comprises three components: self-image, ideal-self and self-esteem (Gross, 2005). Self-image refers to the way in which each individual describes themselves. Ideal-self refers to what kind of a person each individual would like to be and might include appearance and personality. Self-esteem refers to the extent to which one likes, accepts or approves of oneself and how worthwhile one is (Oliver, 1993). Self-esteem can be influenced by how other people view us. Within healthcare settings, how patients feel they are viewed by staff caring for them, or how staff feel they are viewed by colleagues and patients, can affect self-esteem. If a person's own standards are met, they develop a sense of pride, have high self-esteem and feel worthy.

Various other factors are involved in the process of socialisation, which can affect a person's perception and promotion of dignity. Culture is dynamic as the values of community change over time. The scenario of Mrs Smith (Reflective activity 2.4) demonstrates the change in perceptions of 'respect' relating to form of address. Help the Aged (2007) highlighted that many older people find themselves routinely addressed by their first names or endearments in hospital, which they perceive as disrespectful. Acceptable dress codes have also changed in UK society. For example, young people may feel comfortable wearing clothing that exposes their underwear, which would previously have been perceived in our society as undignified.

Previous experiences might also influence one's perception of respect and therefore how a person feels that their dignity has been promoted. For example, abuse in childhood or experience of torture at an early age may affect a person's self-belief or self-concept and the perception of how their dignity is promoted in future. Social standing in the community might influence how one sees oneself; for example, a vicar might expect to be addressed as 'Reverend' instead of by their first name or surname. The situation in which a person finds themselves also influences the way they perceive the maintenance or promotion of dignity (Seedhouse, 2000). For example, you might want to be addressed in a different way in different social settings. The healthcare setting, healthcare procedures and the various interactions with healthcare workers affect how attributes of dignity are maintained. Although dignity is important to people across the age range, perceptions of the attributes of dignity may differ between children and adults (*see* Chapter 8).

The '3Ps' model (Royal College of Nursing, 2008) is useful for considering influences on dignity. These relate to: people (patients, relatives and staff), place (care environment, including organisational culture) and process (care activities). Now consider the scenario and questions in Reflective activity 2.5, which relate to a young woman's experience of healthcare in a community setting. The scenario is a real experience, used with permission and pseudonyms. You will notice that although Bethany was having a procedure performed that was exposing and invasive (process), it was not the actual procedure that affected her dignity so much as the care environment (place) and the staff behaviour (people).

Reflective activity 2.5 A community healthcare experience

Bethany is 25 years old and had her first baby (Amy) four months ago. She is on maternity leave from her job for the local council where she works directly with the public. Her employers emphasise 'excellent customer care' and Bethany won her department's customer care award last year. Bethany's appearance is important to her and she is always smart. She was asked to attend her local doctor's surgery for a cervical smear. Only morning appointments can be made for these and she had no one with whom she could leave Amy. She hoped that Amy would sleep in her buggy during the appointment. She wasn't worried about having the smear as she rationalised that it was important to have it done.

Bethany pushed the buggy into the surgery. The receptionist, who was a lot older than Bethany, shouted at her across the waiting room that buggies must be left outside due to 'health and safety'. Bethany found it embarrassing to be shouted at across a crowded waiting room as though she 'was a child' but she did as she was told and then carried Amy into the waiting room. The nurse called her in and Bethany said that she might cancel her appointment as she had had to leave the buggy outside. The nurse was unsympathetic repeating that it was 'health and safety' and she said that Bethany could hold Amy on her chest.

Bethany found it distressing having to hold Amy on her chest during the smear. Amy was now crying and she vomited over Bethany's face and hair. The nurse offered no assistance. Bethany left the surgery feeling very upset about how she had been treated and aware that she now smelt strongly of 'baby sick'. She considered making a complaint but instead she changed the family's registration to a different surgery.

➤ What attributes of dignity might have been important to Bethany?
➤ What influenced these attributes during her visit to the surgery? Consider the 3Ps: people, place and process.

SUMMARY: THE MEANING OF DIGNITY

This section's discussion has illuminated that patients and clients come from varied backgrounds with different values and expectations regarding the maintenance of their dignity. For example, Mrs Smith expected to be addressed by her title and Bethany expected to be spoken to politely and with concern, as she does when working with the public. Healthcare workers have their own values influenced by their upbringing, age and experiences too. Perceptions of dignity may vary according to the situation we find ourselves in. All these factors influence the maintenance and promotion of patients' or clients' dignity. Key points are that:

➤ everyone has a unique and dynamic concept of dignity
➤ although there is no universal definition of dignity, there are commonly identified attributes of dignity through which it is maintained and promoted
➤ each individual perceives these attributes differently, depending on how they perceive the influencing factors
➤ perceptions of dignity are influenced by experiences in healthcare; the care environment, procedures and healthcare workers' behaviour can all affect perceptions of dignity.

CONCLUSION

This chapter has explored the concept of dignity, firstly by guiding you to reflect on your own perceptions of dignity and then through reviewing theoretical perspectives and research findings. We have suggested that dignity can be defined using its attributes so that we can use a practical approach in the care of clients and patients. We have also introduced the 3Ps of people, place and process, which all influence dignity; these are addressed in detail in this book's other chapters. The chapter has set the scene for the exploration of practical issues concerning the concept of dignity and promotion of patient or client dignity in healthcare. In Chapter 3, the concept of dignity is explored from philosophical and professional perspectives, drawing on media portrayals and a range of literature, thus further expanding your understanding of dignity as a concept.

REFERENCES

Ariño-Blasco S, Tadd W, Boix-Ferrer JA (2005) Dignity and older people: the voice of professionals. *Quality in Ageing* 6(1): 30–5.

Baillie L (2007) *A Case Study of Patient Dignity in an Acute Hospital Setting.* Unpublished thesis. London South Bank University.

Baillie L (2009) Patient dignity in an acute hospital setting: a case study. *International Journal of Nursing Studies* 46: 22–36.

Bayer T, Tadd W, Krajcik S (2005) Dignity: the voice of older people. *Quality in Ageing* 6(1): 22–7.

Beauchamp TL (2001) *Philosophical Ethics: an introduction to moral philosophy.* Boston: McGraw-Hill.

Bernick L, Nisan C, Higgins M (2002) Care of the body: maintaining dignity and respect. *Perspectives* 29(4): 17–21.

Blackstone WT (1970) Human rights and human dignity. In: Gotesky R, Laszlo, E (eds) *Human Dignity – This Century and the Next.* New York: Gordon and Breach, pp.3–36.

Chinn PL, Jacobs MK (1983) *Theory and Nursing – A Systematic Approach.* St Louis: CV Mosby.

Chochinov HM, Hack T, McClement S, Kristjanson L, Harlos M (2002) Dignity in the terminally ill: a developing empirical model. *Social Science and Medicine* 54(3): 433–43.

Collins English Dictionary (2003) *Collins English Dictionary – Complete and Unabridged.* Glasgow: Collins.

Coventry M (2006) Care with dignity: a concept analysis. *Journal of Gerontological Nursing* 32(5): 42–8.

Department of Health (2007) *Privacy and Dignity – A report by the Chief Nursing Officer into Mixed Sex Accommodation in Hospitals.* London: Department of Health.

Enes SPD (2003) An exploration of dignity in palliative care. *Palliative Medicine* 17(3): 263–9.

Fenton E, Mitchell T (2002) Growing old with dignity: a concept analysis. *Nursing Older People* 14(4): 19–21.

Griffin-Heslin VL (2005) An analysis of the concept dignity. *Accident and Emergency Nursing* 13(4): 251–7.

Gross R (2005) *The Science of Mind and Behaviour.* London: Hodder Arnold.

Haddock J (1996) Towards further clarification of the concept of dignity. *Journal of Advanced Nursing* 24(5): 924–31.

Help the Aged (2007) *The Challenge of Dignity in Care: upholding the rights of the individual.* London: Help the Aged.

Jacelon CS (2003) The dignity of elders in an acute care hospital. *Qualitative Health Research* 13(4): 543–56.

Jacelon CS, Connelly TW, Brown R, Proulx K, Vo T (2004) A concept analysis of dignity in older adults. *Journal of Advanced Nursing* 48(1): 76–83.

Jacobs BB (2000) Respect for human dignity in nursing: philosophical and practical perspectives. *Canadian Journal of Nursing Research* 32(2): 15–33.

Jacobson N (2007) Dignity and health: a review. *Social Science and Medicine* 64(2): 292–302.

Johnson PRS (1998) An analysis of 'dignity'. *Theoretical Medicine and Bioethics* 19: 337–52.

Kant I (1909) *Kant's Critique of Practical Reason and Other Works on the Theory of Ethics* (6e). London: Longmans.

Kant I (1948) *Groundwork of Metaphysic of Morals* (Translated by Paton HJ). New York: Harper and Row Publishers.

Mairis ED (1994) Concept clarification in professional practice. *Journal of Advanced Nursing* 19(5): 947–53.

Marcel G (1963) *The Existential Background of Human Dignity.* Cambridge, MA: Harvard University Press.

Marley J (2005) A concept analysis of dignity. In: Cutcliffe JR, McKenna, HP (eds) *The Essential Concepts of Nursing.* Edinburgh: Elsevier, Churchill Livingstone, pp.77–91.

Matiti MR (2002) *Patient Dignity in Nursing: a phenomenological study.* Unpublished thesis. University of Huddersfield School of Education and Professional Development.

Nordenfelt L (2003) Dignity of the elderly: an introduction. *Medicine, Health Care and Philosophy* **6**(2): 99–101.

Nordenfelt L, Edgar A (2005) The four notions of dignity. *Quality in Ageing: Policy, Practice and Research* **6**(1): 17–21.

Oliver RW (1993) *Psychology and Healthcare.* London: Baillière Tindall.

Porkony ME (1989) *The Effects of Nursing Care on Human Dignity in Critically Ill Adults.* Dissertation. University of Virginia.

Randers I, Mattiasson A (2004) Autonomy and integrity: upholding older adult patients' dignity. *Journal of Advanced Nursing* **45**(1): 63–71.

Reed P, Smith P, Fletcher M, Bradding A (2003) Promoting the dignity of the child in hospital. *Nursing Ethics* **10**(1): 67–76.

Royal College of Nursing (2008) *Defending Dignity: challenges and opportunities for nurses.* London: Royal College of Nursing.

Seedhouse D (2000) *Practical Nursing Philosophy. The universal ethical code.* Chichester: Wiley.

Seedhouse D, Gallagher A (2002) Undignifying institutions. *Journal of Medical Ethics* **28**: 368–72.

Shotton L, Seedhouse D (1998) Practical dignity in caring. *Nursing Ethics* **5**(3): 246–55.

Social Care Institute for Excellence (2006) *Practice Guide 15. Dignity in Care.* www.scie.org.uk/publications/guides/guide15/index.asp (accessed 8 October 2010).

Stratton D, Tadd W (2005) Dignity and older people: the voice of society. *Quality in Ageing: Policy, Practice and Research* **6**(1): 37–45.

Woogara J (2005) Privacy and dignity of cancer patients: a qualitative study of patients' privacy in UK National Health Service patient care settings. *Journal of Cancer Education* **20**(2): 119–23.

CHAPTER 3

Professional and ethical expectations for dignity in care

Paul Wainwright

INTRODUCTION

Steven Pinker has said that 'The problem is that "dignity" is a squishy, subjective notion, hardly up to the heavyweight moral demands assigned to it' (Pinker, 2008), while Bostrom has argued that the notion of dignity has uncovered a 'winning formula' encompassing 'a general feel-good quality, and a profound vagueness', which enables all to assert their commitment to it but without 'endorsing any particular course of action' (Bostrom, 2008, p.174). Of these attributes, it is perhaps the 'squishyness' or 'profound vagueness' that has created the biggest problem for healthcare professionals, politicians and the media. It suits many to assert their allegiance with the idea of dignity but few have managed to clear away the vagueness.

In this chapter I explore the concept of dignity from the perspective of professional practice and from the expectations of the general public and service users. In doing so, I explore popular understanding of the concept as revealed by the media and everyday use in common language. I then relate this account to the purpose and practice of nursing and explore the implications of our account in terms of our expectations of professionals and the expectations that service users may reasonably have.

LEARNING OUTCOMES

By the end of the chapter you will be able to:
➤ discuss the common language use of the concept of dignity
➤ explore the relationship between common usage and more theoretical accounts
➤ explain two applications of dignity: to the character of the practitioner and to the treatment of others
➤ debate the meaning and relevance of respect
➤ discuss the relationship between dignity and the purpose of nursing as a practice.

DIGNITY IN COMMON LANGUAGE

In common parlance we talk of people having dignity, behaving in a dignified way or upholding the dignity of their office. We may feel we have been placed (or placed ourselves) in an undignified position, like Mr Pooter who 'left the room in silent dignity but caught my foot in the mat' (Grossmith and Grossmith, 1998, p.77) or that we have been treated in an undignified way. We may be accused of being 'on our dignity'. We may treat others with dignity. And we may dignify others by the way in which we treat them. We say things like 'I won't dignify that remark by replying to it . . .', meaning that to respond would give the offending utterance an importance it did not deserve.

Dignity is a favourite word for journalists. Recent examples from London-based newspapers include many comments about the behaviour of people caught up in the recent earthquake in Haiti, of which Reed Lindsay's is typical: '. . . but then I would witness an act of unsolicited kindness or solidarity or perseverance or dignity, and I would be reminded of the spirit and strength of the Haitian people' (Lindsay, 2010). The novelist Hilary Mantel talks of the perils of writing personal memoirs and the difficulty of emerging 'with a scrap of dignity' (Mantel, 2010), while in a more frivolous tone *The Guardian's* Pass Notes column says, of a minor celebrity, that 'she's appearing on Celebrity Big Brother without completely surrendering her dignity' (*The Guardian*, 2010). And on the more serious side of performance, Eric Siblin, discussing the cellist Pabo Casals, quotes the newspaper *Diario de Barcelona* as praising Casals' performance for 'its diction and dignity' (Siblin, 2010).

An editorial in the *Independent on Sunday* gives several examples of people who, the writer claims, personify dignity. They describe Henry Allingham, a First World War veteran who had died recently, saying that there was 'something about the reticence of Mr Allingham that gave him dignity'. They refer also to the broadcaster, the late Walter Kronkite, whose announcement of the death of President John F Kennedy was 'notable for its restraint and dignity' and to Nelson Mandela, 'another man whose dignity has inspired millions' and whose 'public bearing and lack of bitterness were exemplary', arguing that South Africa 'would be in a much worse position today were it not for his moral stature, and the world would be a less hopeful place'. The editorial concludes with the suggestion that what these men have in common is modesty, and their greatness 'moves and inspires us all the more for their restraint and absence of self-advertisement . . . we believe that quiet dignity still commands respect' (*Independent on Sunday*, 2009). Finally, President Obama, in his Nobel Peace Prize acceptance speech, referred to the 'quiet dignity of reformers like Aung Sang Suu Kyi' (Obama, 2009).

The concept of dignity is used in connection with many things. The preceding examples emphasise the dignified behaviour of the individual but in recent times dignity has been particularly applied to the way we treat other people.

Even in death, dignity is important. A British Coroner states that 'Every case is important to somebody, therefore it's important to me . . . each, I would hope, is treated with sincerity and the dignity it deserves' (McGregor, 2010). Media coverage of disasters has resulted in the publication of photographs of the dead and dying, and this presents challenges for photographers and cameramen, with agencies claiming, for example, that they 'do not use pictures that lack dignity' (Gormley, 2010). But it is in the context of healthcare and, in particular, the care of older people that dignity in the treatment of others has received particular attention in recent years. A typical example is that from Wynne (2010), who offers a graphic account of patients who were unable to get out of bed being instructed by nurses to soil themselves instead of being offered bedpans. Wynne suggests that this was 'an obvious assault on dignity and respect'. We thus have two accounts of dignity. On the one hand it is used to refer to the character of the person, the man with quiet dignity, while on the other it is used to refer to the way others are treated, in ways that protect or threaten dignity. This distinction roughly equates to the distinction made by Beyleveld and Brownsword (2001), between dignity as constraint and dignity as empowerment.

A vivid account of dignity in professional roles comes from the novel by Kazuo Ishiguro, *The Remains of the Day*. Ishiguro has his character Mr Stevens, the butler at Darlington Hall, discuss at some length the nature of dignity in the context of 'great butlers'. The (fictional) Hayes Society, a kind of professional body for butlers, describing the necessary characteristics of applicants for positions in great households, asserts that 'the most crucial criterion is that the applicant be possessed of a dignity in keeping with his position' (Ishiguro, 2005, p.33). Ishiguro has Stevens agree, saying that what distinguishes great butlers from those who are just very competent is 'most closely captured by this word "dignity"'. Stevens describes arguments he had with his friend and fellow butler Mr Graham, who felt that this dignity was akin to a woman's beauty 'and it was thus pointless to attempt to analyse it'. Stevens observes that this would mean that 'this "dignity" was something one possessed or did not by a fluke of nature', just as it would be impossible for an ugly woman to try to 'make herself beautiful'. Stevens believed that dignity, at least in the context of butlering, was 'something one can meaningfully strive for throughout one's career' and he described other butlers who he was sure had 'acquired it over many years of self training and the careful absorbing of experience'. Stevens recounts several anecdotes about butlers who demonstrated great dignity, the point being that in each case the butler had behaved impeccably, successfully managing the situation in spite of the great difficulty with which he was confronted.

Stevens' character is deeply flawed, and one would not want to suggest that professional nurses (or any other professionals) should live their lives in the rather extreme way depicted in the novel. However, Ishiguro's account offers several useful pointers as to the nature of professional dignity.

Dignity thus seems to be attached to persons, their positions and their actions. We may feel that we, or others, possess dignity and we may judge that we or others have acted with dignity. We may describe something or someone as possessing dignity or as being dignified and we may describe an action that bestows dignity on something or someone as dignifying. Dignity appears to be inextricably bound up with our identity and the roles we play. However, from Ishiguro's account and the others quoted above, the character of the person is central. The ability 'not to abandon the professional being he inhabits' must be a quality of the person, not a quality of a professional role, even though the role calls for certain qualities, including dignity, in those who would occupy it. Extending this to ordinary life, away from professional practice, one might say of people like Henry Allingham and Aung Sang Suu Kyi that they had or have the ability not to abandon the person they are, the being they inhabit; 'quiet dignity' means having the strength not to be shaken by the unexpected, the difficult or the distressing. Primo Levi, writing about his experiences in the Nazi concentration camps, notes that it takes a brave man to go to his own death with dignity (Levi, 1991); retaining one's dignity in such appalling circumstances does seem the ultimate in courage and moral strength. This focus on the character of the individual and the challenge of remaining dignified in difficult circumstances is one aspect of Beyleveld and Brownsword's (2001) concept of dignity as constraint. Retaining our dignity in the face of difficulties places constraints on our behaviour, requiring that we do not abandon ourselves, do not give in to fear or anger, and so maintain our quiet dignity.

PROFESSIONAL EXPECTATIONS

Professional expectations of dignity appear to be a central concern for nurses throughout the world. The International Council of Nursing (ICN) Code of Ethics states:

> Inherent in nursing is respect for human rights, including cultural rights, the right to life and choice, to dignity and to be treated with respect. Nursing care is respectful of and unrestricted by considerations of age, colour, creed, culture, disability or illness, gender, sexual orientation, nationality, politics, race or social status (ICN, 2006, p.1; Copyright ©2006 by ICN – International Council of Nurses, 3 place Jean-Marteau, 1201 Geneva, Switzerland).

Later in the document the ICN Code also says: 'The nurse, in providing care, ensures that use of technology and scientific advances are compatible with the safety, dignity and rights of people' (p.3). Other codes, such as the Nursing and

Midwifery Council (NMC) in the UK and the American Nurses Association (ANA) in the USA also include strong statements concerning dignity. The ANA Code, for example, says in Provision 1 that nurses should practise 'with compassion and respect for the inherent dignity, worth and uniqueness of every individual . . .' (ANA, 2001), while the NMC Code states: 'You must treat people as individuals and respect their dignity' (NMC, 2008).

These accounts of dignity and others that appear in national and international codes and charters represent Beyleveld and Brownsword's concept of dignity as empowerment. There is a real danger, however, that such approaches may devalue dignity and render it of little use. The tendency to refer to any and every discomfort or mishap as 'undignified' is not helpful. It is never acceptable for nurses to be rude to patients and still less so for them to neglect people or give poor care. But where we used to talk plainly of poor-quality care, of neglect, of poor management, now everything from thoughtless but minor errors to major failures of care are labelled a matter of dignity. It is not clear what is gained by doing this.

PHILOSOPHICAL BASIS FOR DIGNITY

The philosophical grounds for treating people with dignity are contested but several criteria have been offered and these are critiqued elsewhere (for example, Gallagher and Seedhouse, 2002; Gallagher, 2004, 2007; Gallagher *et al*, 2008; Wainwright and Gallagher, 2008). In brief, a plausible summary would be to follow Nordenfelt (2004) and argue that human beings are of intrinsic worth, what Nordenfelt refers to as *Menschenwürde*, that they may also command respect in the light of their moral conduct and their achievements in life, and finally that a distinctive individual identity is both a source of self-respect and sets up some aspects of the grounds on which we should respect others. I take issue with some of the detail of Nordenfelt's analysis (see for example Wainwright and Gallagher, 2008) but I will simply assert here that both *Menschenwürde* and dignity of identity are helpful concepts for nurses, establishing as they do that we should treat all human beings with respect, regardless of any qualitative account of their lives or health status, and that we should demonstrate contextually appropriate respect for individuals, acknowledging individual preferences and offering individualised care.

DIGNITY AS THE BASIS FOR NURSING

At this point I will take a short digression to consider the goals and purpose of nursing. This seems appropriate as, I will argue, our understanding of nursing is very much about the intention that defines the action. The idea of nursing is a common one in everyday speech and is not confined to the professional usage.

'Nurse' and 'nursing' crop up regularly in literature, with, for example, 34 inclusions in the *Oxford Dictionary of Quotations* (Oxford University Press, 1975). Milton's *Comus* speaks of 'Wisdom's . . . best nurse Contemplation', Campbell says 'and if you nurse a flame . . .', and Goldsmith speaks of 'The land of scholars, and the nurse of arms'. Burke, in his *Reflections on the Revolution in France*, says '. . . the nurse of manly sentiment is gone' and Blake in his *Proverbs from Hell* advises us to 'Sooner murder an infant in its cradle than nurse unacted desires'. Field tells us that 'Public schools are the nurseries of all vice and immorality' and Burns speaks of 'our sulky sullen dame . . . nursing her wrath to keep it warm'. There are many examples that refer to the other notions of nursing, as in Shakespeare's baby, mewling and puking at the nurse's breast, and teachers who continue what the nurse began, but this particular selection has been chosen because they better capture the idea of the purpose of nursing, as opposed to the tasks with which it is associated.

From the examples above and from general usage of the words 'nurse' and 'nursing', a shared meaning emerges, which has to do not with specific actions or tasks but with the intention behind those actions or tasks. To say that contemplation is the best nurse of wisdom is to say that contemplation is the best way to develop the quality of wisdom, to nurture and sustain it. To speak of nursing a flame suggests something fragile, which might be extinguished, but which one might want to protect and to keep alight, sheltering it and keeping it burning. Blake's reference to 'unacted desires' also suggests carrying something and not letting it die or be extinguished, while Burns's sullen dame nursing her wrath reminds us that anger, if it is allowed to, may fade away, while an anger that is fed and nurtured, in other words nursed, will continue to burn.

One can imagine other ways in which one might use 'to nurse' as a verb. For example, we might nurse a business through hard times or perhaps, in schoolboy fiction, imagine our hero nursing his crippled aircraft back to base. A child might nurse her doll, or a kitten or other pet. In forestry it is the practice to plant what is called a nurse crop of fast-growing trees to protect and encourage growth in slower-growing species, and young bees, before they go out foraging, spend some time as nurse bees, feeding the developing larvae of the next generation. The shared intention behind all of these applications of the verb 'to nurse' is thus to indicate some means of preserving, nourishing, sustaining, carrying forward, developing, supporting, holding or protecting something, and this something might be a thing, a plant, a creature, an idea, an emotion or an enterprise.

To identify something – call it for the moment a project – as deserving of being nursed and requiring to be nursed implies some recognition of the worth or value of the project and also of its vulnerability, while to undertake to nurse it requires the motivation that comes from a sense of caring about the success of the project because it is recognised as being of worth. Something that is of no consequence will not call forth the motivation required for it to be nurtured and protected, and a worthy project that is flourishing will not require nursing, although it may still require some care, maintenance and protection. So nursing, I would argue, requires the conjunction of three circumstances. It requires that there be some project of a certain worth (or dignity), that this project is vulnerable or at risk of failing to flourish in some way, and that there is someone prepared to engage with the project so as to try to ensure its survival or flourishing.

Nursing as a healthcare profession illustrates this framework quite well. The project that is the focus of the professional nurse, or indeed the lay carer or the individual sufferer himself or herself (we do, after all, frequently nurse ourselves) is the person who is recognised as having some health need or vulnerability. The particular vulnerability will be health related – the presence of some disease process, some pathology, mental distress or something of the sort. The motivation or intention, the desire to nurture and protect the individual sufferer and protect their dignity, comes from two main sources. The first is society, through the mechanism of the state. Countries like the UK that have state-provided healthcare and support a nursing profession do so out of a collective belief that individuals who need healthcare should be provided with it. The provision of healthcare for all, free at the point of need, is not entirely altruistic – it is to the wider benefit of society that the population is healthy – but clearly rests in part on a belief in the individual worth or dignity of the people who make up that society.

The second factor in the provision of nursing is the character of those who nurse – the individuals who care. It is unfashionable to talk about nursing as a vocation in the religious sense, but there can be no doubt, from the pronouncements of professional regulatory bodies such as the NMC in the UK, that there are clear requirements for nurses to be of a certain character. To become a nurse is to become a certain kind of person, with certain values, attitudes and beliefs.

To nurse in the full sense, to pursue the purpose of nursing as understood from the common language examples above, requires not just the willingness but the desire on the part of the practitioner to engage with people, with a view to nurturing them and pursuing their flourishing and promoting their dignity. Why should both society and individual practitioners desire this? For society and for individual practitioners to invest so much in nursing requires the recognition of something in those who need nursing to call forth the caring response. This, I would argue, is the recognition of the intrinsic worth of human beings, which we might otherwise call human dignity.

WORTH, DIGNITY AND RESPECT

If we equate dignity with worth, then to say that something or someone has dignity is to say they have worth. And to acknowledge worth is to acknowledge that we should treat the worthy object with appropriate respect. The important questions then are: on what grounds do we decide whether a thing has worth or dignity, and, in the event that we decide that it does, how then we should respond. From a nursing perspective, the discussion has mostly focused on the dignity of the individual person and, not surprisingly, the person of the patient. The majority of references to dignity in the healthcare literature and the popular press relate to the way in which patients (in particular vulnerable older people, the dying and the dead) are treated by nurses and by the health-care system in general, and whether and to what extent they are treated with respect.

What amounts to contextually appropriate respectful conduct towards others is, of course, also contentious. Gallagher offers a more detailed discussion of this that draws from the work of Joseph Raz (Raz, 2001; Gallagher, 2007). For Raz, the most basic level of respect involves 'appropriate psychological acknowledgement of value, that is, regarding objects in ways consistent with their value' (Raz, 2001, p.161). Raz argues that there is 'a general reason that if we think of an object which is of value, we should think of it in ways consistent with its value' (p.161). Thus, from a nursing perspective, if we accept the basic premise that all human beings are of fundamental worth, then we should think of them in ways consistent with that worth. Similarly, if we think that a person's individual identity, their preferences and so on, are of value, we should also think of those in ways that are consistent with that value.

Raz suggests a second level of respect, arguing that there is also 'a general reason to preserve what is of value', the strength of that reason varying with the value of the object. As Raz says (p.162), 'we have reason not to destroy, and furthermore, to preserve what is of value'. Thus, Raz's argument supports our earlier analysis of the ordinary language view of nursing: we take steps to nurture, preserve and protect those things that we find to be of value, and we take those appropriately in the context of their value and their need for preservation. We informally nurse our projects and we formally create professional nursing and provide nursing services to people with health needs. There are, as Raz acknowledges, some 'difficult questions regarding the nature and limits of these reasons' but we will not attempt to resolve these here.

Merely preserving things of value represents a rather neutral or static approach, suggesting a curator's concern for a collection rather than the more active and progressive nature of nursing, which we might expect to be concerned with the move from vulnerability to well-being. This brings us to the third stage of Raz's analysis, the need for engagement. Engagement requires, according to Raz, attention and discrimination, and would include, for example, 'spending time with friends in ways appropriate to our relationship with them' (p.163). Contrasting this third stage with the previous two, Raz argues that thinking of valuable objects in appropriate ways and preserving them is only a preliminary, while 'value is realised when it is engaged with'. For nursing to achieve its purpose, whether informally when we nurse our favoured projects or more formally when we deliver professional nursing, if we are to realise the worth of our projects or our patients, there is the requirement for engagement, for caring about as well as caring for the object of our nursing.

THE DIGNITY OF A PRACTICE

As we noted above, the main focus in the healthcare literature is on the dignity of people in their experience as patients. However, I want to introduce a further dimension to the debate, which is to consider the value, or worth, or dignity of a practice, specifically the practice of nursing, and of the dignity of the nurse.

To take the idea of the dignity of a practice first, it may seem odd to apply the concept to a socially constructed notion such as that of a practice. For Kolnai, the characteristics of those things that possess dignity include:

> First – the qualities of composure, calmness, restraint, reserve, and emotions or passions subdued and securely controlled without being negated or dissolved . . . Secondly – the qualities of distinctness, delimitation, and distance; of something that conveys the idea of being intangible, invulnerable, inaccessible to destructive or corruptive or subversive interference . . . Thirdly, in consonance therewith, Dignity also tends to connote the features of self-contained serenity, of a certain inward and toned-down but yet translucent and perceptible power of self-assertion . . . With its firm stance and solid immovability, the dignified quietly defies the world (Kolnai, 1976, pp.253–4, reproduced with permission from Cambridge University Press).

As characteristics of a person, we can probably relate to these and recognise them in individuals for whom we have great respect and who we see as being of particular moral worth, very much in line with the examples given at the beginning of this chapter. But can we apply such a description to an inanimate object? Kolnai suggests that:

> The predicates . . . [of dignity] are chiefly applicable to so-called 'human beings', i.e. persons, but . . . not exclusively so: much dignity in this sense seems to me proper to the Cat, and not a little, with however different connotation, to the Bull or the Elephant . . . is not the austere mountainous plateau of Old Castile a dignified landscape . . . ? And, though man-made, cannot works of art (especially of the 'classic' though not exactly 'classicist' type) have a dignity of their own? (Kolnai, 1976, p.254, reproduced with permission from Cambridge University Press).

While it seems reasonable to view animals and inanimate objects as having intrinsic value or worth, they would lack any capacity for morality. While we acknowledge the notion of the fundamental worth of human beings, the dignity of *Menschenwürde*, any notion of the dignity of people beyond this basic intrinsic worth seems typically to be based on the notion of morality. Thus 'the qualities of composure, calmness, restraint, reserve, and emotions or passions subdued and securely controlled without being negated or dissolved' in a person would reflect their moral character, and while 'the austere mountainous plateau of Old Castile' may invoke feelings of calmness in the observer, this must be a projection, rather than any intrinsic quality in the landscape. Calmness is a human quality and judgement.

But a practice is rather different. It is not a kind of mammal, nor is it an inanimate object, nor even a landscape, although it may have some of the characteristics of at least two of these. It is, first and foremost, a human activity and, fundamentally, a moral activity (*see*, for example, MacIntyre, 1985). Practices result in the realisation of goods, and they demand the pursuit of standards of excellence that are themselves definitive of the practice. A practice has a goal or purpose, which is, by definition, a moral purpose, and in this way practices differ from animals and inanimate objects. It is perhaps not stretching the point too far to suggest that the collective intention of its practitioners, together with the other moral characteristics, gives a practice the kind of intrinsic value or worth that we might well call dignity.

One test of this proposition is to consider the kind of response that practices demand from us. When we reflect on the nursing profession, the medical profession, the clergy or the judiciary (or at least on some notion of them as ideal types), or even Mr Stevens's notion of the 'great butlers', we must surely accord them respect. As Kolnai says of the way we should respond to those things that have dignity, our response:

> must bear a close resemblance to our devoted and admiring appreciation of beauty (its 'high' forms at any rate) on the one hand, to our reverent approval of moral goodness (and admiration, say, for heroic virtue) on the other. Dignity commands empathic respect, a reverential mode of response, an 'upward-looking' type of the *pro* attitude: a 'bowing' gesture if I may so call it (Kolnai, 1976, p.252).

Leaving aside modern cynicism, an idealised or aspirational view of a practice as a moral enterprise or a social good would surely qualify for such a response.

It is perhaps rather easier to understand the dignity of nursing and of the nurse as embodied in the practice of the individual. Nordenfelt includes as one of his types of dignity the idea of dignity of merit, which he says accrues from the attainment of some position of status or significance, either by birth or through one's own success. If we accept the brief sketch offered above of the nature of practices, then achieving admission to a professional practice through one's study, success in examinations and acceptance by one's peers, surely represents the type of situation that Nordenfelt would have in mind. But going beyond the mere elevation to the status of registered nurse, which is on the face of it perhaps the kind of position that Raz would suggest we label simply 'social status' rather than as having dignity, the good nurse, the expert practitioner, might well be expected to display the qualities that Kolnai (1976) describes, 'qualities of composure, calmness, restraint, reserve, and emotions or passions subdued and securely controlled without being negated or dissolved'. Like Mr Stevens's great butlers, the good nurse has the '. . . ability not to abandon the professional being [s]he inhabits'. Good nurses are perhaps good 'by virtue of their ability to inhabit their professional role and inhabit it to the utmost; they will not be shaken out by external events, however surprising, alarming or vexing'.

CONCLUSION

Dignity, despite the reservations of some authors, does appear to have some value as a concept for nursing and, indeed, for other healthcare professionals. It does not have a great deal of specificity or precision as an idea but its vagueness or even 'squishyness' is perhaps part of its value. I would argue that dignity is, at least in some respects, regarded as a virtue, but as with all the virtues it therefore requires the application of prudence or wisdom. Our position can thus be summarised as follows:

➤ dignity is best regarded as essentially a moral quality or virtue
➤ it relates to the intrinsic worth of an object, rather than its exchange value
➤ because of its essentially moral nature, it is best applied to humanity and human activity. Other animals and inanimate objects may possess some similar qualities but these are best regarded in the Aristotelian sense, as characteristic, but not fully characteristic, of dignity
➤ human beings have intrinsic worth, and thus dignity, but beyond this minimal qualification it is the quality of human behaviour and the intention underlying that behaviour that determines its dignity
➤ objects that are of value demand respect, and those that have dignity are of moral worth and demand a particularly moral respect
➤ following Raz (2001), we understand three levels of response to objects of worth: acknowledgement; preservation; engagement
➤ the precise nature of our response must be to the particularity of the situation and thus unpredictable in the detail, but predictable in general principle. In this I follow Kolnai (1976), suggesting a style of response that should be similar to our appreciation of beauty and to our approval

of moral goodness and admiration for virtue on the other. As Kolnai says, 'Dignity commands empathic respect, a reverential mode of response, an "upward-looking" type of the pro attitude: a "bowing" gesture. . . '

I argue that there are three classes or categories of objects, in the context of nursing and healthcare, to which dignity is relevant:

➤ the first of these is the patient (client or service user, and all those associated with the patient, including carers, family members and so on). All such people demand our acknowledgement, preservation and engagement, in recognition of their intrinsic worth as human beings and of their individual identity

➤ second, the individual nurse, as a human being, is entitled to respect in terms of basic humanity, individual identity and in recognition of his or her expertise and professional standing. The professional nurse must also behave with dignity, exhibiting the qualities that characterise the good nurse and the good professional life

➤ thirdly, the practice of nursing has moral worth and demands respect. As a moral endeavour, nursing demands acknowledgement, preservation and engagement, but only in so far as this is justified by the preservation of its purpose and the recognition of its excellence.

Put even more simply, I would argue that the concept of dignity can be reduced to the recognition of moral worth and the appropriately respectful response to that worth, in all areas of human life. In the context of professional nursing, this entitles the patient to expect respectful treatment and behaviour from nurses and places the responsibility on the nurse to embody the notion of respect. This suggests that wisdom, respectfulness and dignity itself are core virtues for nursing as a practice.

REFERENCES

American Nurses Association (2001) *Code of Ethics for Nurses*. Silver Spring: American Nurses Association.

Beyleveld D, Brownsword R (2001) *Human Dignity in Bioethics and Biolaw*. Oxford: Oxford University Press.

Bostrom N (2008) Dignity and enhancement. In: *Human Dignity and Bioethics: essays commissioned by the president's council on bioethics*. Washington, DC: The President's Council on Bioethics, pp.173–207.

Gallagher A (2004) Dignity and respect for dignity – two key health professional values: implications for nursing practice. *Nursing Ethics* **11**(6): 587–99.

Gallagher A (2007) The respectful nurse. *Nursing Ethics* **14**(3): 360–71.

Gallagher A, Seedhouse D (2002) Dignity in care: the views of patients and relatives. *Nursing Times* **98**(43): 38–40.

Gallagher A, Li S, Lee D, Wainwright P, Jones IR (2008) Dignity in the care of older people – a review of the theoretical and empirical literature. *BMC Nursing* **7**(11). www.biomedcentral.com/1472-6955/7/11 (accessed 8 October 2010).

Gormley B (2010) I wasn't very charitable. *The Guardian*, 23 January.

Grossmith G, Grossmith W (1998) *Diary of a Nobody*. Oxford: Oxford Paperbacks.

Independent on Sunday (2010) Editorial. *Independent on Sunday*, 19 July.

International Council for Nurses (2006) *Code of Ethics for Nurses*. Geneva: International Council for Nurses.

Ishiguro K (2005) *The Remains of the Day*. London: Faber.

Kolnai A (1976) Dignity. *Philosophy* **51**: 251–71.

Levi P (1991) *If This is a Man*. London: Abacus.

Lindsay R (2010) Spirit and strength will pull Haiti's people through. *The Observer*, 24 January.

MacIntyre A (1985) *After Virtue: a study in moral theory*. London: Duckworth.

Mantel H (2010) A memoir of my former self. *The Guardian*, 23 January.

McGregor J (2010) On coroners' courts. *The Guardian*, 23 January.

Nordenfelt L (2004) The varieties of dignity. *Health Care Analysis* **12**(2): 69–98.

Nursing and Midwifery Council (2008) *The Code: standards of conduct, performance and ethics for nurses and midwives*. London: Nursing and Midwifery Council.

Obama B (2009) *A Just and Lasting Peace*. http://nobelprize.org/nobel_prizes/peace/laureates/2009/obama-lecture_en.html (accessed 8 October 2010).

Oxford University Press (1975) *Oxford Dictionary of Quotations*. Oxford: Oxford University Press.

Pinker S (2008) The stupidity of dignity: conservative bioethics' latest, most dangerous ploy. *The New Republic*, 28 May. http://pinker.wjh.harvard.edu/articles/media/The Stupidity of Dignity.htm (accessed 8 October 2010).

Raz J (2001) *Value, Respect and Attachment*. Cambridge: Cambridge University Press.

Siblin E (2010) How Bach's cello suites changed Eric Siblin's life. *The Guardian*, 16 January.

The Guardian (2010) Pass notes. *The Guardian*, 18 January.

Wainwright P, Gallagher A (2008) On different types of dignity in nursing care: a critique of Nordenfelt. *Nursing Philosophy* **9**: 46–54.

Wynne A (2010) Shortcuts to bad health care. *The Guardian*, 13 January.

CHAPTER 4

Dignity as a policy issue in healthcare

Alistair Hewison

INTRODUCTION

There has been a lot of talk about dignity recently – politicians, charities, even celebrities are talking about it (Cann and Lishman, 2009). Indeed, since 2006 there has been a growing interest in, and concern about, dignity, or rather the lack of it, in care services in the United Kingdom (UK). This has arisen in part from a series of exposés such as the undercover filming for the BBC Panorama programme, which revealed hospital patients being left in pain without medication, nurses failing to respond to people who desperately needed to use the toilet, patients who were unable to eat going hungry, and some patients dying alone and unnoticed (Whyte, 2008). Similarly when summarising a recent report from the Patients Association (Patients Association, 2009), Boseley (2009) concluded that 'vulnerable and elderly' NHS patients were receiving poor-quality care and being denied their basic dignity in hospitals across the UK. This recognition of failure, in maintaining the dignity of clients, has resulted in it being given prominence in recent health policy focused on quality. The *Next Stage Review* (Department of Health [DH], 2008), or the Darzi review as it is generally referred to, named after its author, states:

> Quality of care includes quality of *caring*. This means how personal care is – the compassion, dignity and respect with which patients are treated. It can only be improved by analysing and understanding patient satisfaction with their own experiences [emphasis in the original] (DH, 2008, p.47).

The purpose of this chapter is to examine how patient dignity became a pressing policy issue in the UK, and what the response to this has been. In order to do this, it is necessary to discuss briefly some key aspects of the policy process to demonstrate how dignity came to be placed on the policy agenda. Next the policy action taken to address the 'dignity problem' will be examined, and finally consideration will be given to whether or not progress has been made.

This is not as straightforward a task as might first appear, because not only is the policy process complex, but there is no agreement on the precise definition of dignity in policy terms. However, this serves to underline the importance of exploring this area of policy. The UK health and social care sector is subject to constant scrutiny, review and policy direction. Without an understanding of this context, practitioners may experience difficulty in maintaining clients' dignity, as they will not be aware of how it is expressed in policy terms, what is expected of them as individual clinicians, or the challenges it presents.

LEARNING OUTCOMES

By the end of the chapter you will be able to:
➤ summarise the policy process in healthcare
➤ examine the role of the government, pressure groups and the media in the UK dignity campaign
➤ discuss policy implementation and how this relates to practitioners and clients in the National Health Service (NHS)
➤ identify the organisational and structural challenges affecting the implementation of the dignity policy
➤ review progress to date and consider the implications for future practice.

THE POLICY PROCESS IN HEALTHCARE

Two definitions usefully summarise the policy process and signal the particular aspects of it that need to be explored in more detail if its effects on health services and patient care are to be understood. For example:

> Health policy refers to the laws and directions from governments that seek to affect and to regulate or to supply state-run health care services. In industrial countries health policy is a major area of political interest and public debate (Cox, 2010, p.294; reproduced with permission from Polity Press).

While this characterisation of policy provides a helpful starting point, it does not fully convey its inherent complexity and tangled nature. This is more evident below:

> Policy making is complex; it is a political activity which crosses national borders. Policies can be made by individuals and organisations, as well as by governments and other agencies, and they can be made at a local level, as well as at regional, national and international levels. Policies at local and national levels often emerge from other policies that have been determined at a global level; however, local policy and practice can also influence global policy making (Earle, 2007, p.5; reproduced with permission from Sage Publications).

In view of this, rather than seek an all-encompassing definition, a way of trying to make sense of policy is to approach it as a process made up of a series of stages (*see* Box 4.1).

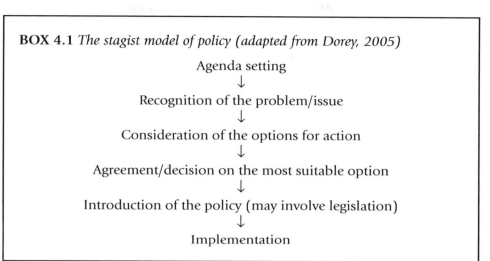

BOX 4.1 *The stagist model of policy (adapted from Dorey, 2005)*

Agenda setting
↓
Recognition of the problem/issue
↓
Consideration of the options for action
↓
Agreement/decision on the most suitable option
↓
Introduction of the policy (may involve legislation)
↓
Implementation

The manifesto of a political party or the underlying ideology of a particular government sets the overall direction for the way it addresses policy issues. For example, the commitment to lower taxation and less public ownership of services such as health and education would result in a distinct policy programme, whereas a party or government with a belief in collective responsibility and the provision of a wide range of public services provided by the state would produce a contrasting set of policies. This overall orientation then influences what are deemed to be 'problems' in need of action. Consequently, unemployment can be a problem, in that it is something that needs to be dealt with. Or it can be perceived as an inevitable consequence of the way the economy works and therefore not requiring attention or specific intervention on the part of government. Once a problem is identified, the options for how best to address it are evaluated, in order to inform a decision about selecting the most effective way of solving it. Finally the policy is put into practice.

Although 'stagist' accounts such as this present an impression of order and logic, this is not accurate by any means. The agenda-setting stage, for example, is not conducted in isolation; it is influenced to a large extent by public opinion and the media (see below). Policy is not always developed in a planned and ordered way; it is often reactive and incremental (Lindblom, 1959, 1979). The use of evidence has been identified as central to the policy process in terms of its design, or 'consideration of options for action'; essentially 'what counts is what works' (Cabinet Office, 1999). However, even when it is agreed that evidence should underpin policy, the availability of different forms of evidence serves to make the process more challenging (Gauld, 2001). In addition, evidence does not provide answers to difficult questions about 'what should be done'; these remain moral and ethical judgements (Greenhalgh and Russell, 2009). Implementation is not a simple act of taking a policy and introducing it, because sometimes the policy is ignored, or more often it is changed by those putting it into practice (Hannigan and Burnard, 2000; Schofield, 2004).

Even this brief review of the stagist model indicates that it is by no means a complete and inclusive account of the policy process. This being the case, why include it here? It is beyond the scope of this chapter to conduct a detailed examination of policy, yet a framework is needed to shape the discussion that follows. So although the stagist model can be called into question for oversimplifying things, it does provide a useful conceptual description of the complex policy process, which breaks it up into manageable parts (Thurber, 2003). With this in mind, the subsequent sections will focus on particular stages of the process as a way of illustrating how dignity became a prominent issue in UK healthcare that demanded action.

GETTING DIGNITY ON THE POLICY AGENDA

If an issue is to appear on the policy agenda, Ham (2004) suggests it must:
➤ attract attention
➤ claim legitimacy
➤ invoke action (Solesbury, 1976; Ham, 2004).

The agenda has been defined as the list of subjects or problems to which government officials, and people outside government closely associated with those officials, are paying some serious attention at any given time (Kingdon, 2003). The 26 departments of the UK government each have more specialised agendas and the key concerns in health are different from those in the Ministry of Justice, for example. Kingdon (2003) offers the useful analogy of a 'policy window' to describe how problems, solutions and decisions come together to generate action. A policy window opens when three streams – problems, proposals and politics – come together. The way these elements came together to raise the profile of dignity in healthcare indicates how an issue that might have been assumed to be a 'given', in the sense that maintaining patients' dignity was a normal and expected part of care, was highlighted as a problem, placed prominently on the policy agenda, and invoked action. The work of Ham (2004) and Kingdon (2003) will be used to inform the explanation of how dignity became a policy issue in healthcare.

Attract attention

In 2006, the Health Care Commission (2006) reported that it found that some older people experienced poor standards of care on general hospital wards, including poorly managed discharges from hospitals, being repeatedly moved from one ward to another for non-clinical reasons, being cared for in mixed-sex bays or wards and having their meals taken away before they could eat them. It recommended that all users of health and social care services should be treated with dignity and respect. This report, along with a series of damning articles in the popular press, such as one in the *Daily Mail* newspaper which estimated that the number of elderly patients starving in NHS wards doubled to 30 000 between 2005 and 2007 (Martin, 2008), all served to ensure that dignity 'attracted attention'.

Claim legitimacy

This issue clearly claimed legitimacy, as it was of interest and concern to politicians and the public. This is reflected in the impetus given to the DH's dignity campaign by a range of bodies and organisations once it was launched. However, in the first instance legitimacy was conferred on this area of policy making through the initiative launched by the Secretary of State for Care Services at the time, Ivan Lewis.

In presenting this policy development, Ivan Lewis acknowledged that health and social care services had made significant progress in reducing waiting times and improving access to services; however, the emphasis on throughput and targets had compromised the quality of patients' experience. The Dignity in Care campaign was aimed at redressing that balance and putting dignity at the heart of care (DH 2006a). Thus, political legitimacy ensured that the need to provide dignity in care would invoke action.

Invoke action

The main way in which action was invoked was through the dignity campaign.

THE DIGNITY IN CARE CAMPAIGN

Formally launched on 14 November 2006, the Dignity in Care campaign (DH, 2006a) was intended to stimulate a national debate around dignity in care, end tolerance of services that did not respect the dignity of those using them and raise the profile of respecting people's dignity. It involved:

➤ the allocation of £67 million to local authorities to enable them to improve the physical environment of care for older people; to help older people living in care homes to do so with dignity; and to enable care homes to be more responsive to the needs of older residents

➤ the issuing of the dignity challenge, a ten-point plan that sets out the national expectations of what constitutes a service that respects dignity (*see* Box 4.2) and the plan to establish a network of local champions of dignity, described as an army of volunteers who would work to raise the profile of dignity in care locally

➤ the issuing of the *Dignity in Care Practice Guide* intended to help frontline staff, practitioners, managers, commissioners, older people and their carers to take up the dignity challenge.

There was also a commitment to review policy in the following areas:
➤ safeguarding vulnerable adults
➤ complaints reforms
➤ training and registration of the workforce
➤ improving the care environment (DH, 2006a).

BOX 4.2 *The dignity challenge (DH, 2006b, 2009a)*

High-quality care services that respect people's dignity should:
1. have a zero tolerance of all forms of abuse
2. support people with the same respect you would want for yourself or a member of your family
3. treat each person as an individual by offering a personalised service
4. enable people to maintain the maximum possible level of independence, choice and control
5. listen and support people to express their needs and wants
6. respect people's right to privacy
7. ensure people feel able to complain without fear of retribution
8. engage with family members and carers as care partners
9. assist people to maintain confidence and a positive self-esteem
10. act to alleviate people's loneliness and isolation.

(Department of Health, 2006b, Crown copyright; reproduced with permission from the Controller of HMSO and the Queen's Printer for Scotland)

It was made clear at the launch that the campaign was not intended to be a 'one-off' event. It was a major priority for the DH and would involve a sustained series of actions, events and policy development (DH, 2006a). This endorsement of the importance of this issue at government level served to cement its legitimacy, and the subsequent programme of events associated with it helped to ensure that sustained action would follow and keep dignity on the policy agenda. For example, two days later (16 November) the Secretary of State wrote to the chairs and chief executives of all the strategic health authorities in England, chairs and chief executives of primary care trusts, chairs of NHS acute trusts and directors of adult social services, amongst others, to explain the campaign and issue the dignity challenge (*see* Box 4.2). He concluded by stating: 'I hope I can count on your support and that together we can create a care system where there is zero tolerance of abuse and disrespect of older people' (DH, 2006b, p.2).

The second major event of the dignity campaign was on 23 January 2007 in Birmingham. The Secretary of State made a speech about dignity, with particular emphasis on the importance of nutrition. During the event he also called on those in attendance to become 'dignity champions', who would challenge bad practice and encourage colleagues and others to look at how dignity can be improved in their locality (DH, 2007a). A dignity champion is someone who believes passionately that being treated with dignity is a basic human right and that care services must be compassionate and person centred, as well as efficient, and are willing to try to help achieve this (DH, 2009a). Examples of such activities include:

➤ challenging disrespectful behaviour
➤ acting as a positive role model by treating other people with respect, particularly those who are less able to stand up for themselves
➤ discussing how to improve the way that services are organised and delivered, in order to maintain dignity
➤ influencing and informing colleagues
➤ listening to and understanding the views and experiences of citizens (DH, 2009b).

Champions are committed to taking action, however small, to create a care system that has compassion and respect for its clients. Each champion's role varies depending on their knowledge, influence and the type of work they do. They include health and social care managers and frontline staff. They also include doctors, dieticians, porters, care workers in care homes, Members of Parliament (MPs), councillors, members of local action groups and local involvement networks (LINks), people from voluntary and advocacy organisations, people who use care services and their relatives and carers as well as members of the public (DH, 2009b).

The campaign is supported by the Royal College of Nursing (RCN), the British Geriatrics Society and Help the Aged, and was boosted by the recruitment of veteran broadcaster Sir Michael Parkinson as its Dignity Ambassador in July 2008. He reported how his mother was starved of care and compassion in a range of establishments leading up to her death, and how this fostered his desire to change the attitude of the NHS and British society to old people (Parkinson, 2008a). He expressed his pride in becoming the ambassador for the campaign that aims to put dignity and respect back at the heart of care by giving a voice to those who need care and encouraging them to stand up and tackle services that do not respect dignity (Parkinson, 2008b). The support of the organisations listed above, and media coverage of further high-profile events such as the National Dignity Tour (BBC, 2008; *Health Service Journal*, 2008) are examples of how the issue continued to be highlighted and helped to ensure that it remained on the policy agenda.

IMPLEMENTING POLICY

As a result of the DH's Dignity in Care campaign, there is no shortage of guidance indicating what practitioners, and indeed all those working in health and social care, need to do to maintain the dignity of clients. For example, guides have been produced by a number of organisations, including Age Concern (2008), the Royal College of Nursing (2008a,b), the Nursing and Midwifery Council (NMC, 2009), and the Social Care Institute for Excellence (SCIE, 2009). This illustrates how charitable bodies, professional regulatory bodies and professional organisations all seek to shape the formation and implementation of policy. They provide detailed instruction and 'best practice' examples to demonstrate how dignity can be delivered. The advice provided is founded on particular definitions of dignity, which are examined in detail in Chapter 2; however, in policy terms, consideration needs to be given to what happens next. Policy can be regarded as both a statement of intent by those seeking to change or control behaviour, and a negotiated output emerging from the implementation process (Barrett, 2004). In practice, this means that putting policy into action often takes place through informal networks and contacts between people rather than through the mechanisms of formal institutions (Newman, 2002). The individual actions of those working in care environments are key to determining whether clients are looked after in a way that promotes and maintains their dignity. However, as in other areas of policy, the success or failure of implementation is affected by a range of factors including the organisational context, leadership, and resources.

CHALLENGES IN IMPLEMENTING DIGNITY POLICY

Two challenges practitioners face in implementing policy related to dignity will be examined briefly to illustrate how policy is of direct relevance to those delivering care. These are the environment of care and working practices.

The environment of care

One of the factors that presents a particular challenge in relation to dignity is the nature of the care environment. The importance of accommodation in the maintenance of patient dignity is examined in Chapter 5; consequently, the focus here is on how action to improve the care environment is being driven by the DH, and in particular the measures being put in place to address the issue of mixed-sex accommodation. This is necessary because in a study involving 2000 interviews with members of the general public, two-thirds of the respondents reported that mixed-sex accommodation was unacceptable because it led to a lack of privacy (DH, 2007b).

Recent policy guidance has made it clear that men and women should not have to share sleeping accommodation or toilet facilities, and from 2010 to

2011 hospitals that fail to achieve this will face serious financial consequences, unless there is an overriding clinical justification (DH, 2010). To help ensure that this target is achieved, an allocation of £100 million has been made to strategic health authorities in England in the form of a privacy and dignity fund which must be used to make the changes in buildings and processes necessary to comply with this requirement (DH, 2009c). Delivery against the privacy and dignity fund plans is being monitored fortnightly, and payment will be withheld if satisfactory progress is not being made (DH, 2009d). This will be managed using 'rigorous and transparent performance measures' from April 2010, to ensure same-sex accommodation is provided for every NHS patient (DH, 2009e). This combination of incentives and penalties is intended to ensure that the sensitive issue of mixed-sex accommodation is addressed and so taken off the policy agenda. However, this can be regarded as 'work in progress' and in the meantime nurses may have to care for people in wards or departments that make it difficult to maintain patients' dignity. Yet the potentially adverse effects of unsuitable surroundings can be offset to a large extent by the actions of those delivering care. The most important consideration for people concerning their privacy and dignity is the attitudes of staff. The seemingly small acts, such as ensuring curtains are completely drawn and toilet doors are closed, have a real impact on the extent to which people feel they have been treated with dignity and respect (DH, 2007b). Chapter 6 considers in detail how staff behaviour can promote dignity.

The NMC (2009) guide states that part of the nurse's responsibility is ensuring that older people are cared for in single-sex accommodation whenever possible (p.12), although it is conceded that 'you may have to work in an environment which is not conducive to delivering care which meets the specific needs of older people' (p.32). In addition, a list of practical actions has been developed by the Chief Nurse to guide nurses in maintaining dignity (Box 4.3).

Now carry out Reflective activity 4.1.

Reflective activity 4.1

As an implementer of policy how can you ensure you comply with the Chief Nurse's list of practical actions (*see* Box 4.3)?

Working practices

The way that care work is carried out is another element of implementation that needs to be considered if the policy commitment to ensure that clients are treated with dignity is to be met. Few conditions are more important than continence with regard to privacy and dignity (Wagg *et al*, 2006), and so data extracts from a recent research report examining privacy and dignity in this

---

BOX 4.3 *The Chief Nurse's advice on dignity (DH, 2007c)*

Practical actions at individual level

➤ Give as much control as possible to patients, for example:
   - do not enter closed curtains unannounced
   - ask patients how they wish to be addressed
   - try to offer a choice of single-sex room or bay if available
➤ Challenge poor practice
➤ Consider becoming a dignity champion
➤ Apologise for every episode of mixing
➤ Give extra personal nursing support to patients in mixed bays, for example:
   - use a separate quiet room for personal conversations
   - avoid giving personal care (for example, toileting) in the bay where possible
   - allocate extra nursing time to confused patients who may act inappropriately.

---

area will be used to illustrate how conflicting working practices need to be balanced by practitioners to maintain clients' dignity. A total of ten individual semi-structured interviews were conducted as part of a broader observational study, seven with nursing home residents and three with hospital patients aged 68–89 years (Billings *et al*, 2009). It is not possible to examine the findings in detail here; however, two brief accounts from the participants are presented as a means of illustrating how different demands in relation to working practices need to be managed by those providing care.

> I mean some people have to be hoisted to the toilet, well I'd hate that. That's what happened when I went into [. . .] hospital for the two weeks, they hoisted me everywhere and boy did I get sick and tired of that. . . . They took all your dignity away. Well as they say you've got no dignity left, I said "No, all the dignity's gone, stand up, pull your pants down, pull them up when you get up" (NH3:4:v3:p.19).

> No. There wouldn't be a choice. The reason is that the hoist is in constant use with other patients and trying to get hold of it is very difficult and I think if you wanted the bed pan, invariably that means that you need to go so they're quite quick with it and they don't hang about, they might take 5 minutes or maybe 10 but there is not a choice, you only get the hoist if you have already got it and you make the opportunity of it. It's not a toilet requisite if you like, it's not, "we'll hoist him out and he can go to the toilet", that doesn't happen (H2:15:V1:p.19).

There is a requirement that all healthcare workers discharge their duty to use machinery and equipment, such as handling aids, where it has been provided for the employee in accordance with the training and/or instruction provided (Health and Safety Executive, 1992). However, in the incidents recorded above, the use of the hoist was implicated in reducing clients' dignity, either because they thought its use undignified or its limited availability presented a risk in relation to safe transfer to the toilet. There is no simple answer here, as both sets of requirements must be met. Safety and dignity need to be maintained. If the potential for a clash between the two competing local policies of maintaining client safety and dignity is to be reduced, then care staff need to deploy a range of skills and knowledge. The RCN (2008b) guide for unit managers, ward managers and team leaders is intended to provide practical support for those wanting to promote and maintain dignity in the workplace. Key to this is 'influence' and 'understanding your organisation' (RCN, 2008a,b). In essence, this requires that practitioners learn more about how their organisations work and seek to influence those around them to focus on dignity as a priority in care. In the situation outlined above, it would involve working closely with clients to build agreement about how best to balance these care priorities in an acceptable manner. In the context of policy implementation, this further emphasises the observation others have made that those delivering services can have a significant effect on how policy is put into practice (Barrett, 2004; Schofield, 2004). Getting results from a policy depends to some degree on the manner in which professionals interpret the policy and incorporate it into their day-to-day work (Barton, 2008), which serves to underline how the different elements of the policy process need to fit together if change is to occur. In the case of dignity, a high-profile media campaign has ensured it is prominent on the policy agenda; support and direction from senior politicians and a range of other organisations have combined to ensure that it claims legitimacy, and those same organisations along with health workers are in the process of invoking action.

PROGRESS

Examination of selected issues in the context of the policy process sheds light on the nature of the challenges involved in ensuring that dignity for clients is managed effectively in a large and complex care service. In this final section, the way these challenges have been addressed will be discussed to evaluate progress. The DH's Dignity in Care campaign has been supported by an investment of £2.5 million and has involved 11 events including conferences, four ministerial 'web-chats', award ceremonies and stakeholder lunches, attended by the Dignity Ambassador. Many resources have also been produced to promote and support the dignity champions (DH, 2009d). In October 2008 it was announced that the 3000th person had volunteered to become a dignity champion (Health4Media, 2008), and by 11 November 2009 the number had risen to 10 000 (DH, 2009f). The success of the campaign has raised the profile of dignity as an issue, and this has been reflected in the emergence of reports charting how initiatives to address dignity issues have improved care.

For example, as part of an initiative conducted between 2007 and 2008 in a district general hospital in Surrey, a series of awareness-raising workshops were undertaken, a bay area in a ward was designated solely for the care of female trauma patients with dementia, and a working group was convened to develop practice further, in order to enhance the privacy and dignity of patients with dementia (Haak, 2009). Elsewhere, staff and patient involvement in the creative arts has been used as a way of exploring and improving shared understandings of dignity (Webster *et al*, 2009 – *see* Chapter 16, 'Enabling dignity in care through practice development'). Finally, Maxwell and Sigsworth (2009) explain how a judgement of non-compliance against the Care Quality Commission's standard on privacy and dignity (20b) stimulated a £10m trust-wide capital redevelopment programme to ensure that the physical environment was changed to improve privacy and dignity in the trust. The project also resulted in a complete culture change, with the maintenance of privacy and dignity being regarded in the same terms as other performance targets.

These examples demonstrate how policy action at a national, organisational and departmental level is needed if it is to be successfully introduced. The challenge for the future will be to ensure it remains on the agenda and does not get sidelined by other pressing issues.

CONCLUSION

Without an understanding of how policy works and an awareness of the influence it has on practice, it is difficult for healthcare workers to bring about change in their organisations. Despite all the high-level activity noted earlier, what dignity means in practical terms can be lost (Cann and Lishman, 2009). Ultimately it is the actions of health and social care staff working with clients that will determine whether or not people are cared for in a dignified manner. If the risk of it becoming a 'buzzword' (Cann and Lishman, 2009) is to be averted, then a continuing and concerted effort is required at every level of policy making to ensure that dignity is kept on the 'agenda'. As Cann (2008) concludes: 'Dignity must not become the victim of political slogans – a concept that everyone agrees is important but no one quite knows how to deliver' (p.2).

REFERENCES

Age Concern (2008) *Quality not Inequality: Age Concern's vision for the future of quality social care.* London: Age Concern.

Barrett SM (2004) Implementation studies: time for a revival? Personal reflections on 20 years of implementation studies. *Public Administration* **82**(2): 249–62.

Barton A (2008) New Labour's management, audit and 'what works' approach to controlling 'untrustworthy' professions. *Public Policy and Administration* **23**(3): 263–77.

BBC News (2008) *Parkinson in Dignity Campaign.* http://news.bbc.co.uk/1/hi/health/7410034.stm (accessed 8 October 2010).

Billings J, Alaszewski H, Wagg A (2009) *Privacy and Dignity in Continence Care Project – attributes of dignified bladder and bowel care in hospital and care homes* (Phase 1 Report). Canterbury: Centre for Health Service Studies, University of Kent/Royal College of Physicians/British Geriatric Society. www.rcplondon.ac.uk/clinical-standards/ceeu/Current-work/Documents/Privacy-and-Dignity-in-Continence-Care-Phase-1-Report-Nov-2009.pdf (accessed 8 October 2010).

Boseley S (2009) Patients 'demeaned' by poor-quality nursing care. *The Guardian* 27 August. www.guardian.co.uk/society/2009/aug/27/patients-association-poor-quality-care (accessed 8 October 2010).

Cabinet Office (1999) *Professional Policy Making for the Twenty-First Century.* London: Cabinet Office.

Cann P (2008) Why does dignity matter? In: *On Our Own Terms: the challenge of assessing dignity in care.* London: The Picker Institute/Help the Aged, p.2.

Cann P, Lishman G (2009) Liberty, equality – and dignity. *Health Service Journal* **119**(6148): 14.

Cox D (2010) Health policy. In: Denny E, Earle S (eds) *Sociology for Nurses* (2e). Cambridge: Polity Press, pp.293–310.

Department of Health (2006a) *£67Million Pledged to Improve Care Homes for Older People.* London: Department of Health. www.mmnetwork.nhs.uk/med-man-new-details.php?newsid=1200 (accessed 8 October 2010).

Department of Health (2006b) *Dignity in Care.* Gateway Reference 7388. London: Department of Health.

Department of Health (2007a) *Speech by Ivan Lewis MP, Parliamentary Under Secretary of State for Care Services, 23 January 2007: Dignity in Care regional event, Birmingham.* London: Department of Health. www.dh.gov.uk/en/News/Speeches/DH_064793 (accessed 8 October 2010).

Department of Health (2007b) *Public Perceptions of Privacy and Dignity – Research Study conducted for the Department of Health.* London: Department of Health.

Department of Health (2007c) *Privacy and Dignity – A Report by the Chief Nursing Officer into Mixed Sex Accommodation in Hospitals.* London: Department of Health.

Department of Health (2008) *High Quality Care for All: NHS next stage review final report.* London: Department of Health.

Department of Health (2009a) *The Dignity Challenge.* London: Department of Health. www.dh.gov.uk/prod_consum_dh/groups/dh_digitalassets/documents/digitalasset/dh_085105.pdf (accessed 8 October 2010).

Department of Health (2009b) *Dignity in Care. Becoming a champion.* London: Department of Health. www.dignityincare.org.uk/_library/Dignity_in_Care_A5_final.pdf (accessed 8 October 2010).

Department of Health (2009c) *The Story so Far. Delivering same-sex accommodation: a progress report.* London: Department of Health.

Department of Health (2009d) *Chief Nurse's Letter: eliminating mixed sex accommodation.* London: Department of Health.

Department of Health (2009e) *Input Assessment – Dignity in Care Campaign.* London: Department of Health.

Department of Health (2009f) *Sir Michael Parkinson's Dignity Champions Reach 10 000.* London: Department of Health. http://webarchive.nationalarchives.gov.uk/+/www.dh.gov.uk/en/MediaCentre/Pressreleasesarchive/DH_108178

Department of Health (2010) *Majority of NHS Trusts Declare Same-Sex Accommodation.* www.wired-gov.net/wg/wg-news-1.nsf/0/73BD8A0278835DE6802576F70038C97E?OpenDocument

Dorey P (2005) *Policy Making in Britain: an introduction.* London: Sage Publications.

Earle S (2007) Promoting public health in a global context. In: Lloyd CE, Hansley S, Douglas J, Earle S, Spurr S (eds) *Policy and Practice in Promoting Public Health.* London: Sage Publications/Open University, pp.1–32.

Gauld R (2001) Contextual pressures on health – implications for policy making and service provision. *Policy Studies* **22**(3/4): 167–79.

Greenhalgh T, Russell J (2009) Evidence-based policymaking: a critique. *Perspectives in Biology and Medicine* **52**(2): 304–18.

Haak N (2009) Maintaining privacy and dignity of patients admitted to a District General NHS Trust. In: Shaw T, Sanders K (eds) *Foundation of Nursing Studies Dissemination Series* **5**(2): 1–4.

Ham C (2004) *Health Policy in Britain* (5e). Basingstoke: Palgrave Macmillan.

Hannigan B, Burnard P (2000) Nursing, politics and policy: a response to Clifford. *Nurse Education Today* **20**(7): 519–23.

Health4Media (2008) *Minister of State for Care Services Announces 3000 Dignity Champions.*

Health and Safety Executive (1992) *The Manual Handling Operations Regulations 1992 (as amended) (MHOR).* London: Health and Safety Executive.

Healthcare Commission (2006) *Living Well in Later Life: a review of progress against the National Service Framework for Older People.* London: Commission for Healthcare Audit and Inspection.

Health Service Journal (2008) Ivan Lewis Begins National Dignity Tour. www.hsj.co.uk/ivan-lewis-begins-national-dignity-tour/1374632.article (accessed 8 October 2010).

Kingdon JW (2003) *Agendas, Alternatives and Public Policies* (2e). New York: Longman.

Lindblom CE (1959) The science of 'muddling through'. *Public Administration Review* **19**: 78–88.

Lindblom CE (1979) Still muddling, not yet through. *Public Administration Review* **39**: 517–25.

Martin D (2008) Number of elderly patients starving in NHS wards doubles to 30 000 in two years. *Daily Mail*, 30 July. www.dailymail.co.uk/health/article-1039562/Number-elderly-patients-starving-NHS-wards-doubles-30–000-years.html#ixzz0We1pbpLJ (accessed 8 October 2010).

Maxwell S, Sigsworth J (2009) Eliminating mixed sex accommodation in hospital to improve patient experience. *Nursing Times* **105**(44): 12–14. www.nursingtimes.net/nursing-practice-clinical-research/acute-care/eliminating-mixed-sex-accommodation-in-hospital-to-improve-patient-experience/5008248.article (accessed 8 October 2010).

Newman J (2002) Putting the 'policy' back into social policy. *Social Policy and Society* 1(4): 347–54.

Nursing and Midwifery Council (2009) *Guidance for the Care of Older People*. London: Nursing and Midwifery Council.

Parkinson M (2008a) Parky's quest for the elderly. *The Sun*, 22 May. www.thesun.co.uk/sol/homepage/showbiz/tv/article1194437.ece (accessed 7 November 2008).

Parkinson M (2008b) Michael Parkinson on dignity. *Telegraph*, 20 May. www.telegraph.co.uk/news/uknews/1997085/Michael-Parkinson-on-Dignity.html (accessed 18 December 2008).

Patients Association (2009) *Patients . . . Not Numbers, People . . . Not Statistics*. London: Patients Association.

Royal College of Nursing (2008a) *Defending Dignity – Challenges and Opportunities for Nursing*. London: Royal College of Nursing.

Royal College of Nursing (2008b) *Small Changes Make a Big Difference: how you can influence to deliver dignified care*. London: Royal College of Nursing.

Schofield J (2004) A model of learned implementation. *Public Administration* 82(2): 283–308.

Social Care Institute for Excellence (2009) *SCIE Guide 15: Dignity in Care*. London: Social Care Institute for Excellence. www.scie.org.uk/publications/guides/guide15/index.asp (accessed 8 October 2010).

Solesbury W (1976) The environmental agenda. *Public Administration* 54(Winter): 379–97.

Thurber JA (2003) Foreword. In: Kingdon JW. *Agendas, Alternatives and Public Policies* (2e). New York: Longman.

Wagg A, Peel P, Lowe D, Potter J (2006) *National Audit of Continence Care for Older People*. London: Clinical Effectiveness Unit/Royal College of Physicians. www.rcplondon.ac.uk/clinical-standards/ceeu/Current-work/Documents/GenericHospital2006.pdf (accessed 8 October 2010).

Webster J, Coats E, Noble G (2009) Enabling privacy and dignity in care: using creative arts to develop practice with older people. In: Sanders K, Shaw T (eds) *Foundation of Nursing Studies Dissemination Series* 5(3): 1–4.

Whyte A (2008) What is going on? *Nursing Standard* 13(22): 18–22.

CHAPTER 5

Care environments that support dignity in care

Ann Gallagher

INTRODUCTION

Care activities are conducted in many different environments, for example, in hospitals, residential homes, patients' own homes, in ambulances and in prisons. Within these environments there is the potential to both develop and diminish dignity. This chapter discusses the meaning and contribution of the care environment to dignity in care. Two aspects of the care environment will be the focus of discussion: the physical care environment and other aspects of the organisation. Some of the concerns relating to undignifying care environments will be examined and examples of good practice discussed. It is concluded that reflection on, and improvements to, the care environment make a significant contribution to patients, relatives and staff feeling valued and respected.

LEARNING OUTCOMES

By the end of this chapter you will be able to:
➤ define the care environment
➤ identify factors that promote dignity in the care environment
➤ identify factors that diminish dignity in the care environment, learning from examples of care environment failings
➤ critically reflect on dignifying and undignifying aspects of one's own care environment
➤ work with colleagues to develop strategies supporting dignity in the care environment.

CARE ENVIRONMENTS

An understanding of the nature and scope of the 'care environment' is a necessary precursor to a discussion of factors that support or diminish dignity. We can think of the environment in narrower and broader terms. As I write, I might think of my immediate environment – the computer, table and sunlight streaming through the window. Or I might think of the wider environment – other buildings in my area, trees, the local town, country and the global context I live within. My environmental concerns may therefore be local and parochial and global. Care environments can also be thought of in more and less limited terms. A healthcare professional may think of the care environment as the immediate area within which he or she delivers care, that is, the bedspace, the outpatients' clinical room or the bathroom. However, for patients, relatives and staff, it is likely that the impact of a care environment will be experienced in relation to the people they encounter, the reception area, cafeterias, and corridors to areas where they receive treatment and care or within which they work.

The scientist Albert Einstein is quoted as saying 'The environment is everything that isn't me' (*see* http://quotationsbook.com/quote/27957). This helpfully reminds us that the environment includes all aspects of our surroundings and includes both people and places. We are, of course, part of the environment of others. The 'care environment' can be defined, therefore, as all aspects of people's surroundings wherein care is received or delivered.

It becomes clear that there are, therefore, many opportunities and challenges regarding the promotion of dignity in the care environment. The reception area and receptionist, for example, have the potential to make patients and families feel welcomed and respected or a nuisance and an inconvenience. Hospital corridors and waiting areas have the potential to make patients and staff feel that they are worthwhile and deserving of cleanliness and comfortable surroundings or, alternatively, disrespected.

Recent reports from United Kingdom (UK) inspection and investigative bodies support the view that there is room for improvement in relation to dignity in care environments. The 13th and final report from the Mental Health Act Commission (2009), for example, detailed environmental conditions reported by commissioners and patients within mental healthcare environments:

> There is use of strong bedding and blankets on the unit, but the blanket had not been washed regularly and there was no bedding between the patient and the plastic mattress. The patient was also not given a pillow to use and had to use her slippers as a make-shift pillow (Mental Health Act Commission, 2009, p.12; reproduced with permission from the Stationery Office).

There were also examples of undignifying care environment conditions in the Patients Association (2009) report *Patients . . . Not Numbers, People . . .Not Statistics*. Ron Kirk's account of his father's experience is as follows:

> Toilets were not cleaned properly with faeces clearly left from several previous uses. My sister often had to clean them herself before she'd let my father use them. My father's swallowing wasn't safe because of his stroke but drinks of

orange juice and water were supplied when the counter instruction over the bed was nil by mouth. We saw dirty and bloodstained food trays. We saw soiled and dirty linen left on floors and mixed with fresh supplies. Personal items for his own comfort frequently went missing (Patients Association, 2009, p.10; reproduced with permission from the Patients Association).

Other relatives reported broken equipment, dirty and uncaring hospital environments, lack of responses to patient needs and requests and moving patients to other wards without consultation. *The Final Report of The Independent Inquiry Into Care Provided by Mid Staffordshire NHS Foundation Trust* (Francis, 2010) was introduced by inquiry chairman, Robert Francis QC, as follows:

I heard so many stories of shocking care . . . The Inquiry found that a chronic shortage of staff, particularly nursing staff, was largely responsible for the substandard care. Morale at the Trust was low, and while many staff did their best in difficult circumstances, others showed a disturbing lack of compassion towards their patients. Staff who spoke out felt ignored and there is strong evidence that many were deterred from doing so through fear and bullying (Francis, 2010, Crown copyright; reproduced with permission from the Controller of HMSO and the Queen's Printer for Scotland).

One example of the 'shocking care' described by Francis is from the wife of a 67-year-old patient. She recalled that call bells were rarely answered and in any case were frequently placed out of reach of patients. She documented that her husband:

. . . soiled his bed time and time again because no-one had answered the call-buttons. On numerous occasions when I arrived on the ward, he was lying in faeces and several times he had been lying in it so long that it dried and caked onto him. Time and again I had to fetch the necessary equipment from the sluice and attend to him myself because there was no staff in evidence on the ward (Francis, 2010, p.392, Crown copyright; reproduced with permission from the Controller of HMSO and the Queen's Printer for Scotland).

These examples are indeed shocking and may be taken to support a view that the UK healthcare system diminishes rather than enhances patient and staff dignity. It is essential to try to understand why these bad experiences come about and why care environments become uncaring and undignifying. There are indications and suggestions within the reports above as to why these situations arise. The Francis (2010) report, for example, identifies low staffing levels, low morale and staff fears of speaking out about poor practice. He also pointed to the impact of a trust making financial cuts when staffing levels were already inadequate. What is evident from this and other reports regarding dignity failings in care environments is that it is rarely the case that the failing is due to an individual but rather a mix of *micro-level, meso-level* and *macro-level* factors.

The Royal College of Nursing report (RCN, 2008) outlines what is meant by each of these levels. The *micro-level* relates to the role of individual responsibility and accountability. Individual healthcare workers should take advantage of opportunities to learn about dignity in care, to be aware of the impact of role modelling and to develop strategies with patients and colleagues that develop dignity in care environments. The RCN survey revealed that almost 80% of nurses left practice feeling that they were unable to deliver dignifying care. It is suggested that this inability is due to organisational (*meso-level*) constraints such as the lack of human and material resources such as equipment and laundry. The *macro-level* factors are attributed to the role of government policy in targets that may diminish dignity in care environments. The lack of progress with single-sex care environments and waiting-time targets would be two examples (RCN, 2008; *see* Chapter 4 for an analysis of health policy relating to single-sex accommodation). The point that staff need to keep the focus on patients was also emphasised by Robert Francis QC (2010):

> People must always come before numbers. Individual patients and their families are what really matters. Statistics, benchmarks and action plans are tools not ends in themselves. They should not come before patients and their experiences. This is what must be remembered by all those who design and implement policy for the NHS (Francis, 2010, p.1, Crown copyright; reproduced with permission from the Controller of HMSO and the Queen's Printer for Scotland).

Thus far it may seem that there is little to celebrate regarding dignity in care environments. There is much scope for improvement but there is also much good practice. A recent RCN evaluation of the impact of a dignity in care campaign (Baillie and Gallagher, 2008) provided many examples of nurse-led initiatives supporting dignity in very diverse care environments.

The 2008 RCN report *Defending Dignity – Challenges and Opportunities for Nursing* distinguishes between two aspects of the care environment – the physical environment and other aspects of the employing organisation. The physical environment has three themes:

1. aspects of the environment maintaining informational and physical privacy (for example, curtains, screens and private spaces for consultation)
2. aesthetic aspects of the physical environment (for example, colour, space, furnishings, décor and music)
3. the provision of single-sex accommodation.

Other aspects of the employing organisation include:

➤ staff attitudes, awareness and knowledge

> ➤ leadership and role modelling
> ➤ teamwork
> ➤ resources (human and material)
> ➤ organisational culture and philosophy.

Focusing on composite vignettes drawn from previous research and practice experience, the next section explores aspects of the physical environment.

DIGNITY AND THE PHYSICAL ENVIRONMENT

The physical environment has the potential to enhance or diminish the dignity of patients and staff. In the previous section, there was consideration of examples of undignifying aspects of the care environment. The examples here (Box 5.1 and Box 5.2) suggest how opportunities to promote dignity in care environments might be maximised.

BOX 5.1 *Vignette 1*

Martha lives alone and finds that she has become increasingly forgetful. She is embarrassed about this and her family are concerned. Her general practitioner has suggested to Martha and her family that she should consider an assessment at the local memory clinic as this may be a form of dementia. Martha is not keen to follow this advice, saying she prefers to retain her independence. After a fall when she is out shopping, she is taken to the accident and emergency (A&E) department at the local hospital. She is not badly hurt but is fearful and appears confused. One of the A&E team (Jean) has expertise in dementia and takes Martha from the curtained A&E area to a quiet room. The room is clean and comfortable and there is a clearly marked toilet nearby. Jean makes Martha a cup of tea and asks her who she would like to be contacted. She contacts Martha's daughter with her consent. Jean spends time with Martha and her daughter talking through support options such as community services and local day centres. Martha admits to feeling lonely and fearful at times and says she would welcome the opportunity to meet other people and to have support to remain at home.

These two vignettes suggest some of the aspects of the physical environment that are likely to develop dignity. In relation to Martha's experience, it seems that Jean was sensitive to her needs and vulnerability. Given her embarrassment regarding her memory lapses and confusion, it seems likely that conducting an interview behind a curtain would not be ideal. She may have had

---

BOX 5.2 *Vignette 2*

Roshan manages a busy acute mental health unit. He was aware that space is limited on the unit and that staff did not have a coffee room or area to store their belongings. One of the rooms had been used as a store-room for another ward. Roshan negotiated an alternative space on an adjoining ward and arranged for the store-room to be converted to a staff room. He presented a case for resources to the unit manager and argued that this initiative supports dignity at work. The manager was sympathetic and allocated a modest budget for the work. Roshan involved staff in selecting the colour scheme and furniture. He also ensured that there is space on the corridor notice-board for the 'staff member of the month' notice.

---

physical privacy (if, that is, the curtains closed properly and people did not intrude) but would not have had informational or auditory privacy as conversations can be overheard. A quiet room is likely to have been more peaceful and private. It is also significant that Jean was able to take time to talk with Martha and her daughter and to offer information about a range of appropriate services. The A&E department at Southampton University Hospitals NHS Trust has such an initiative (Nuffield Council on Bioethics, 2009, p.53). Members of a team, based in the A&E department, provide specialist assistance to people with dementia. It should not be assumed, of course, that Martha has dementia as there may be other explanations for her memory deficits and confusion. However, it is important that she is taken seriously and offered an assessment and appropriate interventions that are respectful of her dignity. The fact that the private room is comfortable and clean is also significant in terms of a dignifying environment.

The second vignette (Box 5.2) relates to dignity at work and suggests how a creative manager might advocate for staff, contributing to their feeling valued by the organisation they work for. Having a notice-board with staff awards is part of the physical environment and also relates to other aspects of organisations.

DIGNITY AND OTHER ASPECTS OF THE ORGANISATION

The RCN report (2008) identified other aspects of the care environment with the potential to enhance or diminish dignity. These include leadership and role modelling, team working, resources and organisational philosophy and culture. Good leadership and 'forward thinking management' were identified as contributory factors to dignifying care (RCN, 2008, p.24). Leaders and managers need, therefore, to act as dignity-promoting role models, being seen, as it were, to 'walk the talk'. Examples of good practice include matrons who accompany ward staff to walk around their ward on a 'stop-and-look' programme. This initiative allows staff to scrutinise their practice area from the perspectives of patients and family members (RCN, 2008; Gallagher *et al*, 2009).

It is suggested that ethical leadership, supporting dignity and other values, may be promoted in at least three ways (Gallagher and Tschudin, 2009). First, having a critical and multidisciplinary approach to professional practice involves learning from the social sciences and public reports detailing and explaining good and poor practice. The Bristol Inquiry, for example, highlighted flawed behaviour, lack of insight, inadequate leadership and 'a club culture' as contributing to unethical practice (Kennedy, 2001). Observing the dignity-promoting practice of others involves reflection on, and learning from, the behaviour and approach of others. Inviting feedback on one's own practice and providing constructive feedback to colleagues are also helpful strategies to promote dignity-promoting leadership. This requires a team ethos and organisational culture that is supportive, open and trusting. The third approach is to provide opportunities for practitioners to develop particular dispositions or virtues such as care, respectfulness, integrity and professional wisdom (Banks and Gallagher, 2009).

A culture of openness where constructive feedback is invited and welcomed is a component of a dignifying organisation echoed in the RCN report. One respondent stated that:

> We work as a supportive team, where mistakes are not judged but used as opportunities to learn. We try to be open about our failures and seek help from each other constantly. We encourage our patients to do the same. If our patients can see where things can improve, we want to know (Staff Nurse, NHS Trust, Acute Hospital) (RCN, 2008, p.25; reproduced with permission from the Royal College of Nursing).

The philosophy of care and website of a healthcare organisation also have the potential to support dignity in care, making explicit the values and priorities of that organisation.

The vignette in Box 5.3 suggests how these aspects of the care environment might support dignity in care.

Features of this vignette illustrate many examples of good practice regarding dignity in care environments. The RCN (2008) report, for example, emphasised the importance of leadership and of leaders role modelling dignifying care. Blake ward appears to be an area where the dignity of both patients and staff is taken seriously. Views may differ regarding the recognition of staff who demonstrate an exceptional ability to deliver dignifying care. Staff recognition awards

---

Box 5.3 *Vignette 3*

The members of staff on Blake ward are proud of the standards of care they deliver. They describe themselves as a supportive multicultural team with strong leadership. The 'team', they say, includes everyone, from the ward clerk and housekeeper to nurses, doctors and porters. The ward manager works alongside new members of staff, students and healthcare assistants, demonstrating, by her example, how to enhance dignity in care. Although the ward does not have single rooms, staff members insist on single-sex sleeping and bathroom areas. A peg and privacy sign is attached to curtains to prevent colleagues inadvertently barging in when an intimate care procedure is under way. The team use the Essence of Care as dignity benchmarks and also meet regularly for dignity training and discussion. Staff, patients and relatives are invited to nominate a staff member for the monthly 'dignity in care' awards. Staff members are encouraged to disclose 'near misses' and to report any aspect of the care environment that appears to compromise dignity in care. All staff members are encouraged to make suggestions as to how to enhance dignity.

---

was one initiative reported in the RCN dignity evaluation (Baillie and Gallagher, 2008). There is evidence that staff may fear the consequences of reporting near misses, errors or poor practice. This suggests that there needs to be a culture where such reporting is commended rather than criticised, and viewed as a learning opportunity rather than as disloyalty. In conducting the RCN dignity evaluation (Baillie and Gallagher, 2008), the author was made aware of many dignity initiatives that resulted from staff members being encouraged to make suggestions as to how to enhance dignity. Examples included an initiative to make the dining room in a nursing home 'more like a restaurant', with napkins and matching tablecloths and with disposable 'bibs' replaced with linen clothes protectors. Other examples included improvements in privacy, with occupied/unoccupied signs on bathroom doors, pegs to hold curtains together and curtains inside toilet doors to prevent exposure.

PRACTICAL APPLICATION

In Chapter 2, you were introduced to the idea that dignity in care is promoted or diminished by people, place and processes. This chapter has focused on *place* in terms of the physical care environment and other aspects of the organisation. The discussion has focused on care in inpatient environments. Healthcare professionals do, of course, deliver care in very different environments including patients' homes, ambulances and prisons. Much of the discussion is transferable to other care environments; however, there will be additional challenges and opportunities. It is, therefore, important that readers reflect on and think creatively about dignity in relation to their own particular environment, taking all who spend time in that environment into account. The focus has been on patients and staff members; however, the dignity of students and visitors should also be considered. In Section 2 of this book, there are chapters considering specific care environments and how they interact with dignity in care.

To apply learning from this chapter to one's own practice it may be helpful to work through Reflective activity 5.1.

Reflective activity 5.1

➤ What does the care environment I work within consist of? Is there, for example, a reception or waiting area, sitting room, staff room, patients' own home?

➤ What aspects of the care environment could be improved regarding dignity in care?

➤ How might these areas be improved, for example, cleanliness, comfort, choice, taking more time?

➤ Who do I need to influence to bring about the necessary change?

➤ If I confront obstacles to the necessary practice change, who might I recruit as allies, for example, other health professionals, managers, patient and carer groups?

➤ How can I evaluate the effectiveness of the change, for example, patient and staff satisfaction?

CONCLUSION

This chapter has explored the relationship between the care environment and dignity. Readers have had the opportunity to reflect on the meaning of the care environment. Examples from reports detailing failings in organisations resulting in patient and staff dignity being compromised were discussed and the importance of appreciating the interrelationship amongst micro-level, meso-level and macro-level factors. Factors that promote and diminish dignity in care environments have been discussed and vignettes providing illustrations have been included. It is hoped that the discussion and reflective questions enable readers to perceive and respond effectively and creatively to dignity deficits in the care environment.

REFERENCES

Baillie L, Gallagher A (2008) *Evaluation of the Royal College of Nursing's 'Dignity at the Heart of Everything We Do' Campaign – The Little Things Make a Difference.* Unpublished report for the RCN.

Banks S, Gallagher, A (2009) *Ethics in Professional Life: virtues for health and social care.* Basingstoke: Palgrave Macmillan.

Francis R (2010) *Final Report of The Independent Inquiry Into Care Provided By Mid Staffordshire NHS Foundation Trust.* http://midstaffsinquiry.com/pressrelease.html (accessed 8 October 2010).

Gallagher A, Tschudin V (2009) Educating for ethical leadership. *Nurse Education Today* **30**(3): 224–7.

Gallagher A, Wainwright P, Baillie L, Ford P (2009) The RCN Dignity Survey: implications for leaders. *Nursing Management* **16**(4): 12–16.

Kennedy I (2001) *The Report of the Public Inquiry into Children's Heart Surgery at the Bristol Royal Infirmary 1984–1995.* CM5207(I). London: The Stationery Office. www.bristol-inquiry.org.uk/final_report/the_report.pdf (accessed 8 October 2010).

Mental Health Act Commission (2009) *Coercion and Consent: monitoring the Mental Health Act 2007–2009 Thirteenth Biennial Report.* London: The Stationery Office.

Nuffield Council on Bioethics (2009) *Dementia: ethical issues.* London: Nuffield Council on Bioethics.

Patients Association (2009) *Patients . . . Not Numbers, People . . . Not Statistics.* London: The Patients Association.

Royal College of Nursing (2008) *Defending Dignity – Challenges and Opportunities for Nursing.* London: RCN.

CHAPTER 6

Staff behaviour and attitudes that promote dignity in care

Lesley Baillie

INTRODUCTION

Staff behaviour and attitudes have a major influence on whether patients experience dignity in care; indeed, Widäng and Fridlund (2003) argued that promoting dignity is *dependent* on how patients are treated by their caregivers. In my doctoral research (Baillie, 2007), a patient who had had major surgery described a nurse who cared for him and maintained his dignity as being:

> . . . sensitive, explains what she's going to do before she does it, she's cheerful, she has a sense of humour, she appears interested in me as an individual, she has a caring approach, appears to enjoy her work – doesn't appear as though it's a chore (Baillie, 2007, p.206).

Clearly the nurse's attitude underpinned her behaviour and approach to care. Other studies have also highlighted the impact of staff attitude on dignity-promoting behaviour. Nåden and Eriksson (2004) found that nurses who promoted dignity had a strong moral attitude underpinned by values such as respect, honesty and responsibility; such nurses had a 'genuine interest and desire to help patients' (p.90). In a study by Bayer *et al* (2005), older people considered that attitudes of caregivers were central to dignified care, as they can portray that the person is valued. In the Royal College of Nursing (RCN, 2008) survey, nurse respondents considered that attitudes of staff themselves particularly influenced the delivery of dignified care. Humanistic caring approaches have been found to promote dignity: treating patients as human beings (Enes, 2003) and holistically (Widäng and Fridlund, 2003) and conveying a caring attitude (McClement *et al*, 2004). Walsh and Kowanko (2002) identified that patients wanted to be acknowledged as a 'living, thinking and experiencing human being not just an object' (p.149).

This chapter explores how staff behaviour and attitudes affect patients' dignity, with a particular focus on communication, privacy and quality fundamental care. The chapter also considers how organisational culture affects individual staff behaviour and how staff should respond when colleagues compromise dignity through their behaviour. The chapter draws on international research findings illuminating the impact of staff behaviour on patients' dignity. Throughout this chapter, for simplicity, the term 'patient' is used, although it is acknowledged that in some care settings the term 'client', 'resident', 'service user' or another term may be more appropriate.

LEARNING OUTCOMES

By the end of the chapter you will be able to:
➤ explain the types of staff behaviour that can diminish patients' dignity
➤ discuss how staff behaviour can promote dignity for patients
➤ analyse how organisational culture can affect individual staff behaviour
➤ consider responses to colleagues' behaviour that compromises patients' dignity.

BEHAVIOUR THAT DIMINISHES THE DIGNITY OF PATIENTS AND CLIENTS

Unfortunately, many reports that refer to loss of dignity suggest that staff behaviour plays a major role. As Chapter 5 explained, the physical care environment and resources also affect dignity but healthcare professionals must acknowledge that their own behaviour and that of their colleagues is highly influential.

Staff behaviour that diminishes dignity is essentially that which is uncaring, as uncaring behaviour from others affects how people feel and whether they feel valued as human beings. Arman and Rehnsfeldt's (2007) study led them to conclude that an uncaring approach was demonstrated when patients were not viewed as 'whole human beings' and caregivers did not recognise their 'existential suffering' (p.373).

Halldorsdottir (1991) highlighted the vulnerability of patients who experienced uncaring. She found that dependent people who felt uncared for felt a sense of loss and dehumanisation, feeling that they had no value as a person: 'an object': 'I was ... a piece of dust on the floor'. In the United Kingdom (UK) in 2009, the Patients Association published *Patients . . . Not Numbers, People . . . Not Statistics*, which provided detailed and shocking accounts of patients' experiences of poor hospital care. The report showed many deficits of management, systems and the care environment, including poor staffing levels, but these reports also referred to individual staff behaviour and attitudes that diminished patients' dignity, including poor communication, and failure to provide pain relief and personal care.

Staff behaviour and attitudes diminish the dignity of patients when they breach privacy, display poor communication and attitudes and deliver inadequate fundamental care. These behaviours clearly contravene professional codes of conduct, legislation and health policies yet continue to be reported.

The UK's Healthcare Commission (2007, p.14) reported on the dignity of older people in hospital and listed 11 categories of commonly received complaints about dignity compromises. Notably, most categories arose from staff behaviour (inappropriate form of address, being spoken about as though the person is not there, not being properly informed, not seeking consent or having wishes considered, being exposed, being left in soiled clothes, lack of help with eating and drinking, being left in pain, abuse and violence). Only a few categories resulted from deficits in the care environment (mixed-sex accommodation, lack of sleep due to noise at night, lack of cleanliness, lack of protection for people's own property, for example, hearing aids). Reflective activity 6.1 relates to the Healthcare Commission's findings.

Reflective activity 6.1 Compromises of dignity

Re-read the previous paragraph: consider the Healthcare Commission's examples of compromises of dignity and reflect on practice in your setting:

➤ have you or your colleagues ever behaved in any of these ways?
➤ if you have observed any of these compromises, what did you do in response?

This chapter later discusses how staff can respond when colleagues compromise patients' dignity.

PROVIDING PRIVACY

Many studies in diverse settings have highlighted that staff behaviour that ensures privacy for patients helps to promote dignity (McClement *et al*, 2004; Matthews and Callister, 2004; Baillie, 2009a).This section considers privacy of personal space, privacy of patients' bodies and confidentiality.

Privacy of personal space

Some studies found that in hospital, patients' personal territory, their bedspace and locker, was not respected by staff (Matiti, 2002; Woogara, 2004). Patients may feel that their personal space has been breached when staff move patients' belongings around in their bedside lockers or other furniture without discussion, or when staff enter closed curtains or doors without asking. Box 6.1 summarises actions to maintain privacy of personal space in different care settings.

BOX 6.1 *How staff can maintain privacy of personal space*

People's own homes

➤ Book appointments in advance (conveys respect and provides people with some control over their own environment).

➤ Knock on the door and introduce yourself, show an identity badge and check the identity of the person answering the door. Explain the purpose of the visit and ask for permission to enter.

➤ Only enter areas of the property necessary for carrying out the care activity, always checking with patients first.

➤ Approach any concerns about their home (for example, safety issues such as lack of heating, trip hazards) constructively and tactfully. Do not make judgemental comments about people's homes.

➤ If using a key to enter a person's home, knock before entering, then call out a greeting and state who you are.

➤ Assess whether to pull curtains, depending on the reason for the visit, the room's position and the potential for people to see in from the street.

➤ Be aware of other people's presence; check discreetly whether the patient wants their relative, friend or neighbour present for support, or whether they would prefer to be alone with you.

Single rooms in care settings

➤ Tell colleagues that you are going to be in a person's room carrying out a procedure, so they will be less likely to enter the room.

➤ Place an 'Engaged' sign on the door as a deterrent to other staff to enter during care delivery or examinations.

➤ Knock before entering and ask whether you can come in. Close the door and cover any window on the door (with the shutters or curtain, as provided) when you are going to carry out care, examine the patient, etc.

➤ Ask first before opening cupboards/drawers to take out items and replace items after use.

➤ Before leaving the room, move any furniture (for example, bed table) back into the position the patient would like and ensure that the person has their call bell.

➤ If possible, negotiate whether the person would like the door left open or shut. N.B. Clinical needs may influence this, for example, infection control, patient safety.

Multi-patient areas (for example, hospital bay)

➤ For personal care, intimate procedures, examinations or private discussions: whenever clinically possible, assist patients out to the toilet, bathroom, treatment or private discussion room, where you can close the door and put on an 'Engaged' sign.

➤ In toilets or bathrooms there may be a 'dignity' curtain inside the door to give added privacy.

➤ Whenever possible, leave patients to use the toilet or shower or bath alone. First assess risk, as some patients will be unsafe to leave alone or might require assistance. Ensure that patients left alone have a call bell.

➤ For patients who are too unwell to leave the bedside or are confined to bed due to their medical condition, explain that their curtains can be pulled whenever needed for privacy.

➤ Apply a clip or a 'do not disturb' notice to the pulled curtain to deter intrusion. Ensure all staff are aware that closed curtains should not be entered by staff without warning.

➤ When pulling curtains, take care that the edges are pulled closely together; report ill-fitting curtains and ask that they are replaced.

➤ If you need to enter the curtains before the patient calls you, ask first if you can enter.

➤ As you enter curtains take care that you do not make a gap so that others can see in.

➤ Show respect for people's belongings and furniture; ask permission before removing items from a locker and before moving furniture.

➤ Ensure that you replace the items where the person would like them and ensure that the person has their call bell.

Privacy of patients' bodies

People undergoing healthcare are at risk of bodily exposure as they often need to undress for procedures or examinations and need help with personal care. Patients may feel that their bodily privacy is violated if they are unnecessarily exposed. Unfortunately, many studies have reported that staff exposed people's bodies and were inattentive to their privacy (Turnock and Kelleher, 2001; Matiti, 2002; Woolhead *et al*, 2005) and that staff intruded behind curtains during intimate procedures involving bodily exposure (Lai and Levy, 2002; Ariño-Blasco *et al*, 2005; Baillie, 2009a). Box 6.2 provides an example of a patient's experience of a breach of privacy in a hospital ward. The patient had a blocked catheter and was having a bladder washout performed when another ward staff member entered the curtains without warning, to talk to the nurse. The patient could not clearly see who had entered the curtains and was acutely aware of his bodily exposure. Not only was his privacy breached but the two staff members talked over him and ignored him. The nurse carrying out the procedure, rather than asking the person to leave and covering the patient, instead engaged in conversation.

> **BOX 6.2** *A breach of privacy during a bladder washout (Baillie, 2007, p.160)*
>
> 'A nurse comes in, draws the curtains round so I'm there, I'm on my back, my frock's [nightshirt's] up round my waist . . . my legs are apart – they've got a bowl in me – and she's syringing me . . . she [another staff member] puts her head through the curtain. Chats to this nurse who's treating me. And I thought – what are you doing – as far as I know, you're not a nurse – you've not come in here for my benefit . . . I felt a bit annoyed. And a bit embarrassed. At the thought that someone who was not medical staff as far as I know . . . I don't know what they were talking about. But it was nothing to do with me. So I got a bit narked. And felt a bit embarrassed. And a certain loss of dignity because I was not in a very dignified position.

Other examples of breach of privacy include bedside curtains that are not fully closed during personal care, removal of clothing without discussion or consent, or providing clothing that does not cover patients' bodies adequately, for example hospital gowns (Baillie, 2009a).

Sometimes, tradition leads to unnecessary bodily exposure, for example patients being expected to undress into nightclothes or hospital gowns long before it is necessary, and for staff convenience, rather than patients' well-being. As well as causing bodily exposure, this practice diminishes dignity by reducing individuality. It also creates a power imbalance between staff who are dressed in uniforms or day clothes, and patients who are dressed in nightwear. Edvardsson's (2008) study highlighted that a person's own clothes were linked with a person's identity; wearing hospital clothing was depersonalising and carried a social stigma. Wilson (2006), in a small project based on a ward for older people, successfully implemented a system to enable patients, where possible, to wear their own day clothes.

Box 6.3 lists ways to minimise indignity resulting from bodily exposure.

> **BOX 6.3** *Minimising indignity caused by bodily exposure*
>
> ➤ Whenever possible, assist patients to dress in their own clothes; if they have to wear nightclothes, provide dressing gowns.
> ➤ In hospitals there are rarely facilities for washing clothes, so do explain this to relatives. Many relatives will agree to bring in nightwear (including a dressing gown and slippers) and day clothes. Ensure that soiled clothing is bagged separately from clean clothing

so it can be taken home for washing, which will help to ensure a constant supply of clean clothing.

➤ When hospital gowns must be used for operations or examinations, ensure that they are fastened properly. There are newer styles available that are less exposing.

➤ Never expect a patient to walk around in a gown without a dressing gown. If there are no dressing gowns available, provide another hospital gown to wear like a dressing gown.

➤ Ensure that patients sitting out in a chair or wheelchair in nightwear or a gown are covered up adequately; for example, use a blanket to cover their legs.

➤ When patients need to undress for procedures or examinations, if they can undress unassisted, leave them to do so unobserved and provide a gown and blanket to cover themselves after undressing.

➤ When you need to expose an area of the patient's body for a procedure or examination, always ask permission first. If possible, ask the patient to move clothing themselves, and only move clothing the minimum amount necessary, ensuring that the rest of the patient's body is covered, by bed linen or clothing. Replace clothing as soon as possible.

➤ Chaperoning (used for protection of both staff and the patient) increases the 'audience', potentially causing further embarrassment for patients. Chaperones should always introduce themselves and give their name and job role. Whenever possible, a chaperone should stand or sit where the patient can see them, and they should talk to the person and avoid looking at their exposed body areas. It is unacceptable for non-healthcare staff (for example, a receptionist) to act as a chaperone.

➤ Some patients will not wish to expose their bodies to staff of the opposite sex, and certain religions may stipulate this requirement. In these situations behave sensitively and ensure that their wishes are respected.

Maintaining confidentiality

Maintaining privacy of information (confidentiality) is another staff behaviour that can promote dignity (Matiti, 2002; Calnan *et al*, 2005). Lack of confidentiality occurs when personal information, for example, about incontinence, medical diagnosis or home circumstances, is overheard or displayed in public areas. Patients are usually well aware that information about them must be shared between healthcare workers to ensure their safety, continuity of care and appropriate referrals. However, information should not be shared unnecessarily between healthcare workers, it should not be shared with patients' families or friends without their permission (except in extreme situations such as an unconscious patient), and patient information must not be shared with other patients, visitors or the media. Most health and social care organisations have confidentiality policies that provide specific guidance about information giving. When families and friends request information about patients, staff should first ask the patient what information they would like to be shared with the enquirer and, if possible, enable them to talk to their relative or friend themselves. In patients' own homes, staff should consider the confidentiality of patients' notes that are left in the home. When information is passed between team members (for example, during a ward round or ward handover), staff should prevent other patients and visitors overhearing. In outpatient areas or waiting rooms, staff should not ask personal questions or carry out procedures, like weighing, in front of other patients.

In curtained areas in hospital, curtains provide a visual barrier but auditory privacy can still be breached. Therefore, taking patients to toilets, bathrooms or a private discussion room is always preferable. When carrying out exposing or intimate procedures at the bedside, staff should communicate discreetly, by keeping voices low and using non-verbal communication. This is particularly important when dealing with personal care, for example incontinence or during an intimate procedure (for example, catheterisation) or examination (for example, vaginal or rectal examination). In a research interview, a patient expressed her embarrassment to me that her consultant spoke so loudly on the ward round that other patients could hear about her urological surgery:

> I just thought, you know "Don't speak too loud" – I'm not exactly proud of what's going on (Baillie, 2007, p.135).

Staff should ensure that patients with hearing impairments have working hearing aids in place and that they can see staff who are talking to them. Potentially embarrassing smells should be dealt with sensitively, by not referring to them verbally or non-verbally and using strategies such as window-opening or sprays quietly and discreetly.

Apart from lack of attention to privacy of the body, there are other forms of behaviour towards people's bodies that can threaten dignity. These include treating people's bodies like objects (Walsh and Kowanko, 2002) and not treating a person's body with respect after death (Söderberg *et al*, 1997).

COMMUNICATION AND ATTITUDES

While privacy is crucial, underlying staff attitudes and values are key to staff behaviour that promotes dignity. Indeed, Applegate and Morse (1994) asserted that privacy-promoting actions such as pulling curtains are of little value if not accompanied by respect for personhood. Similarly, Walsh and Kowanko (2002) concluded that while privacy was important, it was not enough to promote dignity; patients also needed to feel like unique human beings. Women in Widäng *et al*'s (2007) study felt that they were respected when treated as a person, not an object. Staff are more likely to see, and therefore treat, patients as unique human beings if they get to know them; this can be achieved even in acute and short-stay settings through conversation during assessment and essential treatment and care. In care homes for people with dementia, constructing a biography of residents can help caregivers to understand them (Newson, 2008), which should help staff to approach them as individual human beings.

Staff can promote patients' dignity if their interactions help patients to feel comfortable, in control and valued; *see* Box 6.4.

BOX 6.4 *Interactions that help patients to feel comfortable, in control and valued (adapted from Baillie, 2007; RCN, 2008)*

Interactions that help people to feel comfortable
➤ Sensitivity
➤ Empathy
➤ Developing relationships
➤ Conversation
➤ Professionalism
➤ Family involvement (if desired by the patient)
➤ Friendliness and reassurance.
➤ Humour (if used sensitively and appropriately)

Communication that helps people to feel in control
➤ Explanations and information giving
➤ Informed consent
➤ Offering choices and negotiating
➤ Enabling independence

Communication that helps people to feel valued
➤ Listening
➤ Giving time
➤ Showing concern for patients as individuals
➤ Being kind, considerate and helpful
➤ Courtesy: addressing people by their preferred name, introducing self, being polite and respectful, including respect for culture and religious beliefs

---

Now carry out Reflective activity 6.2.

Reflective activity 6.2 Communication to promote dignity

Think back to a recent situation with a patient. You could have been carrying out care or a treatment, investigation or examination. Reflect on the communication that you used during this situation and try to identify specific examples of your verbal and non-verbal communication that might have:

➤ helped the patient to feel comfortable
➤ helped the patient to feel in control
➤ helped the patient to feel valued.

Staff interactions that threaten dignity

Jacobson (2009) focused specifically on behaviours that violated patients' dignity and listed them as rudeness, indifference, condescension (for example, talking down to), dismissal (when practitioners discount patients' concerns, needs, feelings, etc.), disregard (for example, ignoring), dependence (owing to the patient's condition but exacerbated by practitioners' attitudes), intrusion (breaching privacy), objectification (treated as a 'thing' not a person), restriction (of movement, access to belongings), labelling (for example, 'difficult'), contempt (treated without value), discrimination, revulsion, deprivation (for example, preventing access to necessities), assault and abjection (being forced to compromise one's beliefs). Matiti (2002) identified that nurses did not recognise the need for respect to be integral to all procedures, only associating it with personal care. Woogara (2004) reported a general lack of courtesy towards patients, for example, doctors rarely introduced themselves and patients were frequently interrupted by staff while they were eating.

Patients' dignity can be threatened when staff adopt an authoritarian attitude, for example, 'telling' rather than 'asking' patients (Baillie, 2009a). Help the Aged (2007) asserted that talking to older people as though they are children is fairly common, and that endearments like 'sweetheart' or 'darling' may be used rather than an older person's preferred name. Other studies have reported that patients may not be asked how they would like to be called, and first or second names are assumed (Matiti, 2002; Woogara, 2004; Woolhead *et al*, 2005). An interview extract in Goodrich and Cornwell's report (2008) related that during a seven-week stay following a fall, the ambulance crew were the only members of staff who introduced themselves and asked the interviewee's mother how she would like to be addressed. Throughout her hospital stay, staff addressed her mother by her first name, which she had never previously been called by – she had always been called by her middle name. Matiti and Sharman (1999) found that while most patients on a surgical ward preferred first-name terms, some preferred surnames. It is therefore best to ask patients how they wish to be addressed.

More extreme staff behaviour that threatens dignity is inhumane treatment and care (Nordenfelt, 2003). There are reports of staff shouting at patients (Patients' Association, 2009), which could constitute emotional/psychological abuse (World Health Organization, 2002). Abusive behaviour is clearly unacceptable and breaks professional codes of ethics.

QUALITY FUNDAMENTAL CARE

Providing quality fundamental care implies respect and that the person is of value. Examples that have been associated with dignity include ensuring good standards of hygiene and dress (Health Advisory Service [HAS], 2000; Bayer *et al*, 2005), assisting with elimination needs (Calnan *et al*, 2005) and promoting nutrition (Help the Aged, 2007). Textbooks such as Baillie (2009b) detail a caring approach to delivering fundamental care, and UK health policies such as the Essence of Care (NHS Modernisation Agency, 2003) and Fundamentals of Care (Welsh Assembly Government, 2003) set benchmarks for quality fundamental care. Box 6.5 includes two examples of how patients' dignity can be promoted during care activities. Both examples include careful planning, preparing appropriate equipment, thoughtfulness, patient involvement, attention to privacy, and effective communication.

BOX 6.5 *Maintaining dignity during care activities*

Assisting with eating (p.34)

Modified diets are served onto everyday plates; use of the correctly sized spoon or fork; where there is dribbling, the use of a tissue to clean excess; the involvement of the individual in the activity (even in a small way); privacy is offered; verbal interactions with the individual are adult and not infantilising; checking to see that the individual is comfortable with the way that I am 'assisting' them; the individual is offered the opportunity to wash their hands before and after the meal (even if they will play no part in the activity); care is taken to spill no food, but if clothes are soiled, assistance is given to change them (Ward Manager, Acute Hospital).

Bedbath (p.37)

Patient involved in discussion regarding care for the day and is in agreement. Ensure that I have all equipment I require. Ensure I have an assistant to facilitate safe moving and handling. Inform colleagues that I will be undertaking bedbath. Ensure curtains closed. Encourage patient to do as much as they can for themselves during the procedure.

Ensure that only the area being washed is uncovered, that patient is covered and warm throughout procedure. Ensure that patient is involved in conversation. Do not speak about 'what did you do last night' over patient. Offer patient toilet if required. Ensure teeth and mouth clean. Offer drink. Tidy up. Leave patient comfortable with buzzer, drink and ensure that patient has everything they need before leaving them (Practice Development Nurse, Acute Hospital).

(RCN, 2008; used with kind permission from the Royal College of Nursing)

Now carry out Reflective activity 6.3.

Reflective activity 6.3

Consider a care activity or procedure that you regularly carry out in practice. Reflect on how you can carry this out in a way that promotes dignity. Consider careful planning, preparing appropriate equipment, thoughtfulness, patient involvement, attention to privacy, and effective communication.

Inadequate fundamental care

There are many reports of dignity being diminished by staff delivering poor fundamental care; for example, respondents in the Department of Health's (2006) 'Dignity in Care' survey identified lack of assistance with eating, hygiene and elimination. A review of complaints to the Healthcare Commission (2008) included many relating to poor nutrition and hygiene, including patients being left in soiled bedding. Woolhead *et al* (2005) identified a lack of attention to older people's appearance as threatening their dignity. Age Concern's (2006) *Hungry to Be Heard: the scandal of malnourished older people in hospital* described many instances of older people being left hungry in hospital. The Patients' Association (2009) report includes deficits in all aspects of fundamental care, leaving relatives as well as patients devastated. Patients experiencing inadequate fundamental care will feel uncomfortable, uncared for and unvalued as well as experiencing incontinence, hunger, thirst, pain and poor hygiene. All staff should ensure that fundamental care is maintained to a high standard, with privacy and communication that promote dignity.

HOW ORGANISATIONAL CULTURE AFFECTS INDIVIDUAL STAFF BEHAVIOUR

As Chapter 5 explored, organisational culture is influential and includes the social norms of staff and the policies, systems and accepted practices within care settings. Hospital culture can have a positive or a negative effect on how staff behave (Baillie, 2009a). In Walsh and Kowanko's (2002) study, a dehumanising hospital culture was found to diminish the dignity of patients. Conversely, the HAS (2000) study indicated that some wards had a culture of respect for patients and sensitivity to privacy; dignity was highly dependent on the ward manager's leadership.

Staff should reflect on how their own attitudes and behaviour affect patients' dignity but also how these are influenced by institutional culture and their colleagues' behaviour. Each individual staff member should consider how they would respond if colleagues diminish the dignity of patients. In the RCN (2008) nursing workforce survey, respondents reported that other staff, of all disciplines, often breached privacy by entering curtains or rooms without warning. Reflective activity 6.4 explores these issues.

Reflective activity 6.4

➤ How does your organisation's culture influence your attitude and behaviour with patients?

➤ Do you feel that your organisation's culture influences the attitude and behaviour of your colleagues?

➤ How might your own attitude and behaviour towards patients affect those of your colleagues?

➤ What would you do if you observed colleagues displaying attitudes or behaviour that could diminish patients' dignity?

In many cases where abusive behaviour has been uncovered, it has been because of the actions of individual staff members (often junior) speaking out. In the UK, following the 1998 Public Interest Disclosure Act, employees speaking out about malpractice are protected by law, and employers are expected to have whistle-blowing policies (Department of Health, 2003). However, Firth-Cozens *et al*'s survey (2003) identified many barriers to reporting bad practice and that only 56% of nurses reported concerns about practice. They also found that nurses' experiences of reporting bad practice were often negative, highlighting a need for support. Ray (2006) argued that when organisations do not support people who whistle-blow, there is 'a failure of organisational ethics' (p.438). The Healthcare Commission (2008) reported that while 78% of staff said that they would report concerns about negligence or staff wrongdoing, 36% did not know about confidential reporting systems. Organisations must ensure that they have sound systems in place to support staff who report bad practice, and that staff know how to access these.

Box 6.6 makes practical suggestions as to how you could deal with behaviour of colleagues who diminish dignity.

BOX 6.6 *Dealing with colleagues who diminish patients' dignity*

Immediate action

Aim to restore dignity by demonstrating compassion and meeting immediate dignity needs. Some examples:

➤ if a colleague exposes a patient unnecessarily, depending on the situation, cover the patient up, offer a dressing gown or help the patient to dress, pull the curtains fully closed

➤ if a colleague fails to introduce themselves, introduce them to the patient

➤ if a colleague talks over a patient, instead involve the patient in the conversation

➤ offer explanations and information (when they are not offered) and ensure patients' consent and involvement in decisions, where absent

➤ apologise to patients for your colleagues' behaviour, where appropriate.

Speaking to your colleague

➤ Raise the issue in privacy by taking them to a quiet room to discuss.

➤ Focus on their behaviour, not them personally.

➤ Encourage them to reflect on how their behaviour might make the patient feel.

➤ Aim to be constructive: suggest how they can adjust their behaviour to promote rather than diminish dignity.

➤ Where applicable, reinforce any positive behaviour that they showed.

Reporting

➤ If a colleague's behaviour consistently lacks attention to dignity, or an isolated incident was particularly serious, talk to their manager or use your organisation's whistle-blowing policy to report the behaviour.

➤ Document the details of the incident(s), writing clearly exactly what happened and the people involved.

CONCLUSION

Dignity in healthcare is 'everybody's business'; all staff who work with patients, regardless of their qualification and role, have a crucial influence on whether patients' dignity is promoted. Even if the environment is far from ideal, the individual interactions between staff and patients and their families can have a major impact on whether they feel cared for and valued as human beings. Privacy, communication and quality fundamental care are key aspects of staff behaviour that promote dignity in care. Staff should be aware of how organisational culture affects their own behaviour towards patients. They should also be prepared to deal with diminished dignity arising from the behaviour of colleagues, using whistle-blowing policies as necessary.

REFERENCES

Age Concern (2006) *Hungry to Be Heard: the scandal of malnourished older people in hospital.* London: Age Concern.

Applegate M, Morse J (1994) Personal privacy and interaction patterns in a nursing home. *Journal of Ageing Studies* **8**(4): 413–34.

Ariño-Blasco S, Tadd W, Boix-Ferrer JA (2005) Dignity and older people: the voice of professionals. *Quality in Ageing* **6**(1): 30–35.

Arman M, Rehnsfeldt A (2007) The 'little extra' that alleviates suffering. *Nursing Ethics* **14**: 372–86.

Baillie L (2007) *A Case Study of Patient Dignity in an Acute Hospital Setting.* Unpublished thesis. London South Bank University.

Baillie L (2009a) Patient dignity in an acute hospital setting: a case study. *International Journal of Nursing Studies* **46**: 22–36.

Baillie L (2009b) *Developing Practical Adult Nursing Skills* (3e). London: Hodder Arnold.

Bayer T, Tadd W, Krajcik S (2005) Dignity: the voice of older people. *Quality in Ageing* **6**(1): 22–7.

Calnan M, Woolhead G, Dieppe P (2005)Views on dignity in providing health care for older people. *Nursing Times* **101**(33): 38–41.

Department of Health (2003) *Whistle-blowing in the NHS Policy Pack.* London: Department of Health.

Department of Health (2006) *Dignity in Care Public Survey October 2006 – Report of the Survey.* Gateway reference 7213. London: Department of Health. www.dh.gov.uk/prod_consum_dh/groups/dh_digitalassets/@dh/@en/documents/digitalasset/dh_4139558.pdf (accessed 11 October 2010).

Edvardsson D (2008) Balancing between being a person and being a patient – a qualitative study of wearing patient clothing. *International Journal of Nursing Studies* **46**(10): 4–11.

Enes SPD (2003) An exploration of dignity in palliative care. *Palliative Medicine* **17**(3): 263–9.

Firth-Cozens J, Firth RA, Booth S (2003) Attitudes to and experiences of reporting poor care. *Clinical Governance* **8**(4): 331–6.

Goodrich J, Cornwell J (2008) *Seeing the Person in the Patient.* London: King's Fund.

Halldorsdottir S (1991) Five basic modes of being with another. In: Gaut DA, Leininger MM (eds) *Caring: the compassionate healer.* New York: National League for Nursing Press, pp.37–49.

Health Advisory Service (2000) *'Not Because They are Old': an independent inquiry into the care of older people on acute wards in general hospitals.* London: Health Advisory Service.

Healthcare Commission (2007) *Caring for Dignity: a national report on dignity in care for older people while in hospital.* London: Commission for Healthcare Audit and Inspection.

Healthcare Commission (2008) *Learning from Investigations.* London: Healthcare Commission.

Help the Aged (2007) *The Challenge of Dignity in Care: upholding the rights of the individual.* London: Help the Aged.

Jacobson N (2009) Dignity violation in healthcare. *Qualitative Health Research* **19**(11): 1536–47.

Lai CY, Levy V (2002) Hong Kong Chinese women's experiences of vaginal examinations in labour. *Midwifery* **18**(4): 296–303.

Matiti MR (2002) *Patient Dignity in Nursing: a phenomenological study.* Unpublished thesis. University of Huddersfield School of Education and Professional Development.

Matiti M, Sharman J (1999) Dignity: a study of pre-operative patients. *Nursing Standard* **14**(13–15): 32–35.

Matthews R, Callister LC (2004) Childbearing women's perceptions of nursing care that promotes dignity. *Journal of Obstetrics, Gynaecologic and Neonatal Nursing* **33**(4): 498–507.

McClement SE, Chochinov HM, Hack T *et al* (2004) Dignity-conserving care: application of research findings to practice. *International Journal of Palliative Care* **10**(4): 173–9.

Nåden D, Eriksson K (2004) Understanding the importance of values and moral attitudes in nursing care in preserving human dignity. *Nursing Science Quarterly* **17**(1): 86–91.

Newson P (2008) Dignified care for staff and residents. *Nursing and Residential Care* **10**(1): 608–13.

NHS Modernisation Agency (2003) *Essence of Care: patient-focused benchmarks for clinical governance.* London: NHS Modernisation Agency.

Nordenfelt L (2003) Dignity of the elderly: an introduction. *Medicine, Health Care and Philosophy* **6**(2): 99–101.

Patients Association (2009) *Patients . . . Not Numbers, People . . . Not Statistics.* London: Patients Association.

Ray SL (2006) Whistleblowing and organisational ethics. *Nursing Ethics* **13**: 438–45.

Royal College of Nursing (2008) *Defending Dignity: challenges and opportunities for nurses.* London: Royal College of Nursing.

Söderberg A, Gilje F, Norberg A (1997) Dignity in situations of ethical difficulty in intensive care. *Intensive and Critical Care Nursing* **13**(3): 135–44.

Turnock C, Kelleher M (2001) Maintaining patient dignity in intensive care settings. *Intensive and Critical Care Nursing* **17**(3): 144–54.

Walsh K, Kowanko I (2002) Nurses' and patients' perceptions of dignity. *International Journal of Nursing Practice* **8**(3): 143–51.

Welsh Assembly Government (2003) *Fundamentals of Care: guidance for health and social care staff.* Cardiff: Welsh Assembly.

Widäng I, Fridlund B (2003) Self-respect, dignity and confidence: conceptions of integrity among male patients. *Journal of Advanced Nursing* **42**(1): 47–56.

Widäng I, Fridlund B, Martenssen J (2007) Women patients' conceptions of integrity within health care: a phenomenographic study. *Journal of Advanced Nursing* **61**(5): 540–8.

Wilson D (2006) Giving patients a choice of what to wear in hospital. *Nursing Times* **102**(20): 29–31.

Woogara J (2004) *Patient Privacy: an ethnographic study of privacy in NHS patient settings.* Unpublished PhD thesis. University of Surrey.

Woolhead G, Calnan M, Dieppe P, Tadd W (2005) Dignity in older age: what do older people in the United Kingdom think? *Age and Ageing* **33**(2): 165–70.

World Health Organization (2002) *The Toronto Declaration on the Global Prevention of Elder Abuse.* Geneva: World Health Organization.

SECTION 2
Dignity in different healthcare settings

CHAPTER 7

Dignity for children

Paula Reed

INTRODUCTION

In this chapter I discuss dignity in relation to children. For the purposes of this chapter, the term 'children' is used to cover all children and young people from the age of 0 to 16 years. 'Dignity' is a term that is not always associated with children, especially young children and babies. As those who work with children and young people will recognise, there is huge variation of developmental stage including awareness, dependency, abilities and understanding within these ages. In order to address this spectrum I have used three case studies to illustrate some of the issues that are pertinent to this diverse client group: two from the acute hospital setting and one in the community. Dignity campaigns (Department of Health [DH], 2006; Royal College of Nursing, [RCN] 2008) have raised the profile of dignity in care in the United Kingdom (UK) (*see* Chapter 4: 'Dignity as a policy issue in healthcare'), but dignity remains a concept associated with older people rather than a term linked with children. In this chapter, I explore the meaning of dignity for children and demonstrate how dignity-promoting practice is as important for children and their families as for any other group.

I commence by reviewing what is currently understood by dignity and children. I have made particular reference to work undertaken around promoting the rights of the child and their participation in both society and their own healthcare. I will then explore the social construction of children and their position in society, and look at areas in which dignity can be promoted or diminished for children in practice and consider the environment, the processes and the people involved in the care of the child (Gallagher *et al*, 2009). Gallagher *et al* (2009) distil the themes that underpin dignity into: places, people, processes. Important too are the values at the level of society, the institution, for example the hospital, and the individual people involved.

To be able to protect and promote the dignity of children and young people in a range of settings, we need to understand what dignity means when it is linked with young people. It is easy to make assumptions about dignity for children based on what is understood about adult dignity, but is dignity for children the same or different from that of adults? There has been a groundswell of interest in promoting the dignity of older people, particularly in hospital, but there has been limited research on dignity and children. However, recent research has been undertaken to challenge adult-centric assumptions and demonstrated some of the particular aspects of care that affect children's and young people's sense of dignity. Examples in this chapter have been informed by an ethnographic approach to understanding the meanings of dignity for children, their parents and the staff looking after them on a children's ward (Reed *et al*, 2003; Reed, 2007). Ethnography is a useful methodology to tap into the direct experience of participants. In this example, the study involved a nine-month period of fieldwork on a children's ward in a district general hospital. The research took a broad approach to understanding dignity for children, focusing not only on, for example, the need for privacy, but exploring the entirety of the experience of children in hospital or other care settings and linking it back to the impact on the child and their feelings and sense of dignity. The research identified themes central to the promotion of dignity for children. This chapter's case study examples are drawn from my research; all names have been changed to protect confidentiality.

I conclude the chapter with an exploration of the practical application of dignity-promoting practice in child healthcare settings. I have included some questions to encourage reflection on practice and stimulate further discussion. In my final summary, I will draw together the key points covered in this chapter.

LEARNING OUTCOMES

By the end of the chapter you will be able to:
➤ understand some of the issues pertinent to the protection and promotion of dignity for children
➤ identify some of the threats to dignity for babies, children and adolescents
➤ challenge your own beliefs/practices with regard to children and young people.

DIGNITY AND THE CHILD

The inherent dignity of the child is emphasised by the United Nations (UN) Convention of the Rights of the Child (1989). Children should be treated with humanity and respect for the inherent dignity of the human person and in a manner which takes into account the needs of persons of his or her age (Article 37). The rights of disabled children are described in Article 23, which demands that they be able to enjoy a full and decent life, their dignity is ensured, and self-reliance and active participation in the community are promoted. The convention also recognises that by reason of physical and mental immaturity, children need special safeguards and care, with their best interests being the primary consideration. I will discuss some of the challenges to these ideals in caring for children when they are in hospital or cared for in the community and how dignity-promoting care can be delivered in practice.

POWER AND THE CHILD

An acknowledgment of the vulnerability of a child is also the recognition of an imbalance of power between the child and adults. These power relations are built upon the view that childhood is a discrete category of human life (Lloyd-Smith and Tarr, 2000). Balen *et al* (2006) suggest that children are constructed as 'human becomings' rather than human beings in their own right, and that their present is sublimated with their future in mind. There have been recent UK government initiatives to improve outcomes for all children and raise the profile of the well-being of children, for example *Every Child Matters* (Department for Education and Skills, 2004), as well as multi-agency initiatives to increase the participation of children in society and ensuring that children and young people have a strong voice in the development, delivery and evaluation of services that affect their lives (Participation Works Partnership, 2010). Nevertheless, at a societal level, the voices of children remain quiet. Adults assume a considerable degree of power over children and what happens to them. Rather than placing importance on the here and now experiences of children, it has been argued that children are judged, nurtured and protected with the future adult in mind (Christensen, 1998). The child and their childhood matter less.

Powerlessness may be compounded by ill health and admission to hospital. Research with adults indicates that a feeling of powerlessness and loss of control has a negative impact on one's sense of dignity (RCN, 2008). Within a hospital setting, the lives of the children, and to a lesser extent their families, are subjugated to the routines of the hospital. Dignity has been linked with the feeling of being in control and being able to make decisions for ourselves and yet these are feelings that many children and young people lack, especially when they are unwell or hospitalised.

There are individual and socially constructed reasons why children and young people are vulnerable to having their dignity unacknowledged or overlooked. Children are used to adults having control over them; young children are small and can be carried or moved at the whim of the health worker. Young children may not be able to talk or articulate their views and staff may be tempted not to communicate directly to them. Attempts by babies to communicate, such as crying, may not always be listened to by busy staff and staff may communicate with parents but this is not always adequate.

FAMILY-CENTRED CARE

Baillie *et al* (2009) identify the culture of the organisation as influential in promoting the dignity of patients. Central to the care of children and young people is the ideology of family-centred care. This has grown up in recognition of the importance of parental presence and involvement in the way children are cared for when they are ill. The National Service Framework for Children (DH, 2003, 2004) upholds the ideal of care being integrated and coordinated around the particular needs of the child as well as the needs of the family. This trend is based upon the premise of the beneficial influence of the family in the care of children (Corlett and Twycross, 2006).

The ethos of family-centred care has been promoted on children's wards and situates the child within his/her family. Care is planned by health staff around the whole family rather than just the individual child, with the aim of minimising emotional trauma and assisting recovery. Family-centred care has intuitive appeal to health carers and yet there is a lack of evidence to demonstrate that family-centred care improves the child's experience (Shields *et al*, 2007; Carter, 2008). Family-centred care assumes a cohesive family unit. However, at times of stress such as when a child becomes ill, even the closest families can become discordant. Adolescents may naturally be in conflict with parents, and agreeing an approach to care can become very difficult. Coyne (2006) showed that parents were not always able to take part in family-centred care due to other commitments and some resented doing what they considered to be the work of the nurses.

Where family-centred care works, it can promote communication between the parents, child and staff. Parents can advocate for their child and ensure that their needs are met. They can help their child understand about their illness and what is happening as well as providing safe and familiar support. However, the voice of the child and their opinion, especially if it conflicts with the staff, can be lost (Reed, 2007).

Researchers investigating the experiences of children in hospital have drawn attention to the way the desire to protect children, or a paternalistic attitude by healthcare workers, can have the effect of limiting a child's opportunity to express their opinions. Carter (2002), in her discussion of chronic pain, argues that the professional can base their interpretation of a child's pain on clinical experience alone rather than an appreciation of the lived experience of the child. It can be difficult for children to communicate effectively; they may have limited verbal skills due to their condition or their stage of development. There may be opportunities now for children to play in hospital and express themselves in this way, but neither doctors nor nurses are regularly involved in these activities and they are not able to capitalise on these episodes to understand the children more holistically.

Staff and parents may work together in the 'best interests' of the child. Respecting the dignity and experience of a child is fundamental to determining best interest. Promoting the dignity of a child may, in some circumstances, mean challenging the basis on which decisions are made or treatments initiated. Procedures may be undertaken despite the protestations of a child, with the intention of doing what was best, either for the child now or for their future well-being. Carnevale (1997) uses the uncomfortable term 'aggressive care' following his ethnographic research in a paediatric intensive care unit. Children may need to be 'held down' or restrained for procedures. However, where staff are busy and under pressure themselves, clinical expediency can determine their actions. For example, it can be tempting to take blood from a baby before he/she has finished their feed or while they are still asleep. It is important to question for whose best interests we work: the child, the member of staff, or the parent? Sometimes, for the well-being of all the patients on a ward, procedures have to be undertaken at a particular time in order that the staff member can attend to others on the ward. There is always the tension of the needs of another taking priority at ward level; this can threaten an individual's dignity.

Dealing with patients and their parents who challenge the way we work can be difficult. Promoting the dignity of such children and parents can be testing. Equally, parents and their children may be overly compliant and there is evidence to suggest that children and their families do not challenge decisions and practice because they want to keep on the right side of staff. As one mother of a 17-month-old boy explained:

> We are scared of upsetting them, you know. A lot of the time we let things ride because we thought maybe there's a bigger battle round the corner (Reed, 2007, p.288).

In either situation, the best interests of the child may not be achieved.

THE ENVIRONMENT

The importance of the environment in safeguarding the dignity of an individual is widely recognised in the discourse (Coyne, 2006; Baillie *et al*, 2009). Children and young people are cared for in a variety of settings, from acute hospitals, to hospices, in their own homes and in schools. Every setting raises its own particular challenges to the promotion and protection of the dignity of an individual child. The environment is key to putting children at their ease:

> An appropriate, well cared for environment engenders feelings of worth especially among children, young people, their parents and possibly staff (Baillie *et al*, 2009, p.28).

The layout of the ward is important. Many wards now have a play area/room, but if a child has to walk a long way or past the nurse's station then they may be discouraged to go.

In hospital the ward, its layout, the lack of privacy, the bright lights, food and routines are strange to a child and their parents. Those who stay in hospital for up to 48 hours can suspend their normal way of living as if they were just visiting. However, those who must stay in for a prolonged period or who have to return frequently have to live in hospital and adapt their way of living accordingly. Meal times, bed times and the timings of procedures are all taken out of their hands. This can deny them their sense of control and independence; in turn this can undermine their self-esteem and sense of dignity.

Children and young people appreciate comfort and seek out comfort on the ward. Where children are placed in mixed open bays, they have little opportunity to personalise their space around them. In side rooms one can observe the way children and their families will fill the space with their personal effects. Self-expression and identity can be threatened in hospital and yet it is an intrinsic part of both dignity and the young person's personal growth. Lewis *et al* (2009) describe the benefits of using the hospital bedside space to give visual cues to nurses, thereby enabling them to know their patients more intimately and in a way that is more meaningful.

Normality is something that we all crave; particularly in times of stress and distress, we yearn for the familiar and that which is safe. Hospitals and other healthcare settings can be very alien places to children, young people and their parents, in terms of both the physical environment and the sights, sounds and smells they encounter. It can be this very strangeness that threatens the individual's sense of control, ease, self-expression and determination. By acknowledging some of this strangeness and thinking of ways to overcome it, we can go a long way in putting patients and their families at ease, and arguably promote their sense of dignity.

Dignity can be more difficult to maintain where the ward caters for a variety of ages. Older children can find it insulting being put in a bed next to a young child. They can find adhering to early lights out and early rising an additional strain and a disregard for their needs as adolescents. Equally, in wards that have a range of conditions, staff may have more empathy for those children and families who are 'truly' sick with long-term and serious illnesses, and lack compassion for those recovering from routine yet nevertheless painful and upsetting procedures. Equally, parents of children with chronic illness may regard the families of children with minor ailments with disdain and be aware of uninvited interest of other families on the ward.

PRIVACY

There is a considerable body of research to support the idea that the maintenance of privacy is fundamental to the promotion of dignity (Walsh and Kowanko, 2002; Webster and Bryan, 2009). Research indicates that children are perceived by staff and parents to have an increasing sense of bodily privacy, from very little in babies, to an acute sense of bodily privacy in adolescence (Reed, 2007). This growing awareness is thought to be modelled by parents and promoted by staff.

There are some important areas when the privacy of individual children and young people can be undermined. Staff, seeking to promote privacy, adopt stylised behaviours, such as pulling curtains, that demonstrate that dignity is being addressed. However, children do not necessarily recognise these behaviours as such. They may feel more secure with the curtains not closed or they may be particularly sensitive to the crack in the curtain left open, or the reality that sounds and conversations are not kept confidential by curtains alone.

Staff manage the bodies of children throughout their hospital stay, covering exposed bodies, observing, measuring and breaching body boundaries with the insertion of drips and drains. In hospital, the bodies of children are no longer private but become the objects of interest, discussion and examination, with their appearance being the source of speculation and conjecture as to what may be wrong with them. The children and their bodies can become defined by the clinical gaze and medical measurements. Foucault (1973) documents the transformations in medical practice that took place towards the end of the 18th century. He describes the way the body became the new 'anatomical atlas' to be interpreted through the 'clinical gaze'. The role of the patient diminished as the body became the object of study (Williams and Bendelow, 1998). Children who have many or prolonged periods of time in hospital can experience a considerable amount of handling by relative strangers. Staff and even parents can become desensitised to drips and drains and handle them without regard to the sensitivities of the patient. Yet children and young people may be acutely aware of their physical appearance and stigma.

Dignity for children is complex, as the discussion has so far identified. The case study in Box 7.1 raises a few points for discussion; for example, what features of this scenario are pertinent in considering the dignity of the young person involved?

Sometimes, when providing intimate care or undertaking intimate procedures, staff may seem not to react to a potentially embarrassing task. Staff may use behaviours or words to minimise the size, significance or severity of an event. These 'minifisms', suggests Lawler (1991), protect the member of staff and the patient from having to acknowledge and deal with embarrassment. However, Carl (in Box 7.1) found the episode where the female nurse took a swab degrading. Children's developing sexuality is often avoided, yet is an important part of their developing sense of self.

Children develop and redevelop their sense of identity as they grow up. Fundamental to establishing self-identity are the choices we make over the way we present ourselves. Choices for children over presentation of self are very limited

---

BOX 7.1 *Case study A*

Carl was a 14-year-old boy with cystic fibrosis. He had been admitted many times, and on this occasion with an acute infection requiring intravenous antibiotics. He expressed his feelings of humiliation when a nurse, just a few years older than he, took a swab from his groin.

Carl felt ridiculous in a hospital gown and was reprimanded when he wore just boxer shorts on the ward, as they were judged unsuitable. He pulled out a nasogastric tube as he found it stigmatising and sensed that people stared at it.

Carl missed his friends from home. He also commented on how he would make friends with children and young people on the ward and then they would 'disappear' and he would not know how they were unless they were readmitted. He felt that staff did not respect his need for friendships. He resented having to, yet had to put up with their noise early in the morning. Carl longed for normality and felt that the world was passing by, leaving him behind.

Carl's mother had a difficult role to play. She wanted to be there to advocate for her son and yet she was aware that at 14 he did not want to have her around all the time. She felt some of the staff did not like her and thought she interfered. She was not medically trained, yet over the years she had acquired a detailed understanding of cystic fibrosis and thought she had the right and ability to question the staff about the treatments and their care of her son.

---

on a children's ward. Children can be humiliated by being forced to wear clothes that are not their own. Hospital gowns can be particularly disliked by boys who see them as dresses and, rather than devices to protect their dignity, perceive them to be embarrassing. Moreover, children and young people, such as Carl, may be taken from the relative privacy of the ward through more public areas of the hospital dressed in hospital wear with an assortment of drips and drains.

Adolescence is a time of great changes in a young person, both physical and emotional. It is a time characterised by emerging independence and disattachment from the primary caregivers (usually parents). Yet in hospital this natural progression is compromised as parents are frequently resident, spending a great deal of time with their adolescent child, and important friendships and the establishment of peer groups are undermined.

Despite acknowledgement of the dignity of all persons, even the very young (UN, 1989), in practice it can be a difficult notion to appreciate with very young children. Babies are unable to communicate their needs verbally. They are small and unable to move themselves around and their daily needs have to be met through another. This makes them vulnerable to being overlooked in terms of dignity. Reed (2007, p.256) cites the acknowledgment of this vulnerability from a staff nurse:

> They are only babies, so people think it doesn't matter

and later:

> People think "Oh it's a baby we can just go ahead and do it".

The case study in Box 7.2 illustrates privacy issues related to a young child in hospital.

BOX 7.2 *Case study B*

Jaynie was a 21-month-old girl. She had been readmitted with pneumonia for the sixth time and was waiting in the eight-bedded assessment bay to be seen by the registrar. Since birth she had been subjected to a raft of tests, but still a definitive diagnosis had not been made. Privacy was difficult to maintain in this area as it was next to the entrance and held children of all ages and their families prior to admission or discharge home. Jaynie's mother found the attentions of other families painful, and repeatedly telling and retelling her story to different health professionals in such an environment was distressing. Jaynie's routines were disrupted and she had undergone several painful procedures, including a lumbar puncture, during previous admissions.

Autonomy is recognised as important in the preservation of dignity. Indeed, it has been argued that autonomy is a more tangible and useful concept to measure and therefore achieve than the more nebulous notion of dignity (Macklin, 2003). The idea of autonomy for babies and very young children at first seems impossible and inappropriate (Pullman, 1999). Yet autonomy for children the age of Jaynie (*see* Box 7.2) has been described by a mother (Reed, 2007) as the freedom to listen and respond to bodily needs such as sleep and hunger when they need to.

Children and their families are particularly aware of the eyes and ears of the other families on the ward. They are constantly scrutinised not only by staff but by other patients and their families. Darbyshire (1994) described this phenomenon as 'parenting in public'. Parents of disabled children have described their loss of normal parenting and described the transformation of parenting from private to being conducted under the gaze of healthcare workers (Kirk *et al*, 2005). Thus, parents can be upset by the others looking on and even by doctors, where they perceive their interest to be disingenuous, for example, curious about the medical condition rather than the child's well-being.

STAFF–PATIENT RELATIONSHIPS

Research demonstrates that children and their parents appreciate the relationship they develop with the staff (Reed, 2007). However, the position of the trained children's nurse is ever further from the child and their intimate care, leaving limited opportunities for staff on a ward environment to establish relationships. A sense that they were treated with dignity and a feeling that their dignity remained intact were reported to be integral to the relationships between children and their parents and the staff. The style of communication is fundamental to the promotion and protection of an individual (Wainwright, 1994).

Children and their parents want to feel that they matter. They want to be listened to and have their opinions respected. Parents do not want their child objectified but acknowledged as an individual. They want staff to demonstrate interest in their child as people and as individuals, and appreciate it when staff make an effort to get to know them. Children want to be spoken to and not over (Reed, 2007).

Several papers identify communication along with environment as key to the promotion of dignity (RCN, 2008). I have already described some of the issues to be aware of in family-centred care, but there are also other aspects of interaction that are important to consider. One needs to be aware that even if you have seen a child coming in for a routine tonsillectomy or appendectomy, it is the first time for the child, and for many the first time in the strange hospital environment with strange nurses and doctors. Another issue is attention to pace and timing. Sometimes, information is badly received because the timing was wrong and the healthcare professional was communicating within their own timeframe, unaware of the needs of the patient. For example, soon after Jaynie (Box 7.2) was born, a junior doctor came to check her over before discharge, but suggested that she was seen by the registrar first. The registrar had come swiftly over, stating 'I understand that you are worried about Down's', to which Jaynie's parents had replied 'No but we are now'.

Research (Reed, 2007) indicates that some children are likely to receive more attention from staff than others. Teenage girls, for example, are able to establish a rapport readily with the nurses, the majority of whom are female and often not much older. For teenage boys, this relationship can be more awkward, as in Carl's experience. In a general children's ward, children with learning difficulties or mental illness may be avoided by staff and communication may be limited, with parents/carers expected to undertake most of the caring role (Brown and Guvenir, 2008). Stockwell (1972) first identified characteristics of patients who were not popular. Those that received more attention were those with whom staff could develop reciprocity in their relationship.

Children and young people, especially those with chronic health needs, grow up whist undergoing treatment and care. The DH (2003) identified that the changing needs of children were not always considered. Box 7.3 presents an extract from an interview at home with Luke (aged 6 years) and his mother, reminiscing about the tough times they spent together in hospital when Luke was being treated for cancer and had a Hickman line ('Wiggly').

BOX 7.3 *Interview extract (Reed, 2007, p.301)*

Luke (aged 6 years) at home with mum 24 months post treatment.

Mum: 'She used to give him something to drink, didn't she, and then we take out some ketchup'.
Luke: 'It was blood, Mum!'
Mum: 'Oh I am sorry, was it, Luke? We called it ketchup at the time'.

Box 7.3 demonstrates how those in a caring role need to be alert to the developing and maturing child. Ways of communicating and explaining treatments effectively need to be modified as children grow up.

Reflective activity 7.1 presents a list of reflective questions to help you to explore dignity for children and their parents in your care environment.

Reflective activity 7.1

➤ Try entering the ward or the environment in which you work and imagine yourself as a child coming to this place for the first time. What does it smell like, what does it look like, what are the people around you doing, are there other children, how do they seem? What can you hear? How does this make you feel? You can test out your hunches with the children themselves, or their parents.

Consider

➤ How do I feel about this patient (and their parents)? How does this influence my response to them, and in particular my attention to protecting and promoting their dignity?
➤ Are there patients/families that I avoid? Why is this? How does this influence their stay in hospital?
➤ Are there patients I enjoy being with/looking after? How does this affect their dignity?
➤ What activities do I do to promote dignity? Are they working? Do they work in every case?

CONCLUSION

In this chapter I have explored the importance of dignity for children and young people in healthcare. To assume that dignity is of lesser importance for children and young people arguably denies their very humanness and is a reflection of their position in society. At a practical level, there are some particular issues pertaining to children and young people to consider when promoting dignity in healthcare.

I have not provided a 'dignity checklist', but rather drawn attention to some points to consider for best practice when caring for children and young people. I have discussed the impact of the environment in promoting dignity for children, with particular reference to the hospital ward. Particular to the care of children in hospital is the presence of family and family-centred care, which creates its own challenges to maintaining dignity. Linked to the environment is the individual's need for privacy and their parents'/carers' need for privacy and refuge from the scrutiny of fellow patients and staff. Patient confidentiality is fundamental to a relationship between patient and staff, but this can be difficult to maintain on an 'open' ward with the privacy of family life made public. Nursing and medical staff can become desensitised to bodily exposures, and without careful attentiveness can inadvertently cause a patient humiliation and distress. Loss of autonomy and independence has been noted as fundamental to feelings of a loss of dignity in older people; children, by contrast, may be prevented from developing this independence and have their presentation of themselves severely restricted. It should be borne in mind that there is a power differential between the child and an adult, which is compounded by their role of patient. This, combined with barriers to communication, means that questions of best interest must be carefully negotiated.

Paramount to the promotion of dignity is the interaction between the child and the healthcare worker. To engage fully with a child, one must engage with that child's subjective experience. This requires challenging traditional accepted ways of doing things by taking the perspective of the child. Listening to children and communicating using child-friendly methods such as play improve this understanding. Being reflective and aware of one's own attitudes and resultant behaviours can assist human encounters and communication, no matter what the age.

REFERENCES

Baillie L, Ford P, Gallagher A, Wainwright P (2009) Dignified care for children and young people: nurses' perspectives. *Paediatric Nursing* 21(2): 24–8.

Balen R, Blyth E, Calabretto H *et al* (2006) Involving children in health and social research: 'human becomings' or 'active agents.' *Childhood* 13(1): 29–48.

Brown F, Guvenir J (2008) The experiences of children with learning disabilities, their carers and staff during hospital admission. *British Journal of Learning Disabilities* **37**: 110–15.

Carnevale F (1997) The experiences of critically ill children: narratives in the making. *Intensive and Critical Care Nursing* **13**: 49–52.

Carter B (2002) Chronic pain in childhood and the medical encounter: professional ventriloquism and hidden voices. *Qualitative Health Research* **12**: 28–41.

Carter B (2008) Commentary on Shields L, Pratt J, Davis L, Hunter J. Family-centred care: a review of qualitative studies. *Journal of Clinical Nursing* **5**: 1317–1323.

Christensen P (1998) Difference and similarity: how children's competencies are constituted in illness and its treatment. In: Hutchby I, Moran-Ellis J (eds) *Children and Social Competence: arenas of action.* London: Falmer, pp.187–201.

Corlett J, Twycross A (2006) Negotiation of care by children's nurses: lessons from research. *Paediatric Nursing* **18**(8): 34–7.

Coyne I (2006) Children's experiences of hospitalisation. *Journal of Child Health Care* **10**(4): 326–36.

Darbyshire P (1994) *Living with a Sick Child in Hospital: the experiences of parents and nurses.* London: Chapman and Hall.

Department for Education and Skills (2004) *Every Child Matters: change for children.* Nottingham: DfES Publications.

Department of Health (2003) *Getting the Right Start: National Service Framework for Children.* London: Department of Health.

Department of Health (2004) *Children and Young People Who are Ill: National Service Framework for Children, Young People and Maternity Services: standard 6, part II.* London: Department of Health.

Department of Health (2006) *Dignity in Care.* Gateway Reference 7388. London: Department of Health.

Foucault M (1973) *The Birth of the Clinic: an archaeology of medical perception.* Translated from the French by AM Sheridan. London: Tavistock.

Gallagher A, Wainwright P, Baillie L, Ford P (2009) The RCN Dignity Survey: implications for leaders. *Nursing Management* **16**(4): 12–16.

Kirk S, Glendinning C, Callery P (2005) Parent or nurse? The experience of being the parent of a technology dependent child. *Journal of Advanced Nursing* **51**(5): 456–64.

Lawler J (1991) *Behind the Screens: nursing, somology and the problem of the body.* Melbourne, Edinburgh: Churchill Livingstone.

Lewis P, Kerridge I, Jorden CFC (2009) Creating space: hospital bedside displays as facilitators of communication between children and nurses. *Journal of Child Health Care* **13**: 93.

Lloyd-Smith M, Tarr J (2000) Researching children's perspectives: a sociological dimension. In: Lewis A, Lindsay G (eds) *Researching Children's Perspectives.* Buckingham/Philadelphia: Open University Press, pp.59–70.

Macklin R (2003) Dignity is a useless concept. *BMJ* **327**: 1419–20.

Participation Works Partnership (2010) *About us.* www.participationworks.org.uk/about-us (accessed 25 October 2010).

Pullman D (1999) The ethics of autonomy and dignity in long term care. *Canadian Journal of Aging* **18**(1): 26–46.

Reed P (2007) *Dignity and the Child in Hospital.* Unpublished PhD thesis. University of Surrey.

Reed P, Smith P, Fletcher M, Bradding A (2003) Promoting the dignity of the child in hospital. *Nursing Ethics* **10**(1): 67–76.

Royal College of Nursing (2008) *Defending Dignity: opportunities and challenges for nursing.* London: Royal College of Nursing.

Shields L, Pratt J, Davis L, Hunter J (2007) Family-centred care for children in hospital. *Cochrane Database of Systematic Reviews* **1**: CD004811.

Stockwell F (2002) The unpopular patient. In: Rafferty AM, Traynor M (eds) *Exemplary Research for Nursing and Midwifery.* London: Routledge, pp.23–42.

United Nations (1989) *Convention on the Rights of the Child.* www.unicef.org/crc/ (accessed 11 October 2010).

Wainwright P (1994) The observation of intimate aspects of care. In: Hunt G (ed) *Ethical Issues in Nursing.* London and New York: Routledge, pp.38–54.

Walsh K, Kowanko I (2002) Nurses' and patients' perceptions of dignity. *International Journal of Nursing Practice* **8**: 143–51.

Webster C, Bryan K (2009) Older people's views of dignity and how it can be promoted in a hospital environment. *Journal of Clinical Nursing* **18**(12): 1784–92.

Williams S, Bendelow G (1998) *The Lived Body: sociological themes, embodied issues.* London and New York: Routledge.

CHAPTER 8

Dignity in maternity care

Barbara Burden

INTRODUCTION

Ask any midwife about dignity within maternity care and they are likely to tell you the age-old adage that mothers leave it 'at the door to the maternity unit and collect it on the way out'. Over the years that I have practised as a midwife I have found this portrayal of dignity intriguing and somewhat difficult to qualify. The notion of dignity being removed from a person poses a number of questions; for example, what is it about being pregnant that requires mothers to lose or relinquish their dignity? Is this a midwife's perception of what happens to mothers or do mothers acknowledge it as occurring? Can a woman have a baby with dignity? And at what stage in her pregnancy does a mother feel that she has parted with her dignity and, if so, does she get it back and how? These questions became one element within a grounded theory research study on privacy in maternity care environments (Burden, 2007), which explored the perception of privacy and its inherent relationship with dignity, the results of which provide the foundation for this chapter. The case studies and quotations used throughout the chapter are from the research study; all names used are pseudonyms.

LEARNING OUTCOMES

By the end of this chapter you will have:
➤ explored the concept of dignity in relation to privacy in maternity care environments
➤ considered the strategies mothers use in maternity settings to enable them to maintain dignity in childbirth
➤ reviewed how the concepts explored in this chapter relate to your own area of practice.

PRIVACY AND DIGNITY DURING PREGNANCY AND CHILDBIRTH

Privacy and dignity are concepts which, while generically defined, are interpreted by us as individuals. We each have identified boundaries of privacy which, while predominantly unique, have commonalities such as shame, embarrassment and need for respect and solitude (Halmos, 1953; Schneider, 1977; Bloustein, 2003). As individuals we usually have reasonable control over our privacy (Bloustein, 2003) but this can change with the circumstances in which we find ourselves. In the case of pregnant women, these boundaries are influenced by contact with health professionals, the need for health surveillance and the environment of care (Burden, 2007). The outcome is a process of adaptation where mothers attempt to maintain their privacy and dignity by putting in place strategies that enable them to deal with the intimacy involved with the process of childbirth, and then revisit their privacy and dignity after the birth has occurred. These strategies focus upon losing one's inhibitions, solitude and withdrawal, self-introversion, dealing with the indignity of ward-based procedures and losing face in a public environment. The chapter explores all these areas in detail.

The idea of creating new life and delivering a baby into the world is an exciting experience for most mothers; it does result, though, in women being subjected to a range of intimate examinations or processes that, if undertaken at other times, may be perceived as intrusive. During the process of pregnancy, birth and the early postnatal period, mothers find themselves subjected to varying degrees of physical assessments, from abdominal examinations and vaginal examinations to fetal blood sampling or induction of labour. It is the repetitive nature of early examinations that mothers describe as desensitising them to subsequent and more invasive examinations later in their pregnancy and that ultimately concludes with a loss of their inhibitions.

LOSING ONE'S INHIBITIONS

Inhibition can be described as the defence mechanisms or barriers we put in place to protect us from the embarrassment of our actions, or the actions of others, and which in turn impose restraints on our behaviour. For example, some women feel comfortable sunbathing topless on the beach whereas others would not consider exposing themselves so openly in a public place. It is the level of inhibition that we have for a given activity that predicts our level of embarrassment. Therefore, if a mother is happy to expose her breasts in public, the notion of breastfeeding in a public place may not be such an issue for her. Where our level of inhibition is consciously reduced this is mirrored by a subsequent decrease in our levels of embarrassment and shame. This is shown where mothers, as they become accustomed to physical examinations such as abdominal and vaginal examinations, put in place strategies based upon their previous experiences, to manage lowering both their inhibitions and their embarrassment during such interactions.

Women know their boundaries of privacy and dignity in any given situation and are usually able to ensure that their privacy needs are met. As with the development of any experience, privacy status is governed by previous actions and experiences (Goffman, 1963, 1967; Rosen, 2001). It is therefore inevitable that expectant mothers commence their pregnancy with their own unique requirements for privacy and dignity, based on prior experience. Within my study there were mothers who, for example, had never had a cervical smear or a vaginal examination before becoming pregnant, in some cases actively postponing examinations because of the embarrassment and indignity they perceived would result. This meant that some mothers embarked upon pregnancy either with no preconception of what would happen to them during the birth or with a somewhat idealistic view that they would remain in control of their bodily privacy and their dignity during pregnancy. For some mothers this came with a naivety relating to the type and number of examinations they would be subjected to and a view that they could refuse, or keep examinations to a minimum.

Upon entering pregnancy mothers in my study described themselves as 'private in mind and body' and 'shy'. Most mothers had an idealistic view that they would not be admitted to hospital until they were in labour, at which time they would have their own room and their own midwife who would be providing all their care, and would labour with their clothes on. For example, it was only with hindsight that the following two mothers were able to consider how private their bodies were prior to pregnancy and how their privacy and dignity boundaries changed throughout their experience.

> Before I had the baby, I didn't realise it but I was quite a private person . . . Looking back I think, knowing now how private I was, how did I get through that whole experience?

> You go into it [pregnancy] thinking I don't want to show myself at all and I don't really want too many people in the room. I am quite shy and what have you.

Mothers perceive routine examinations to be embedded in the process of pregnancy, as an acknowledgement of both their pregnancy and the need to determine the viability of their baby. They are viewed as something over which they have little control if they want a successful outcome to their pregnancy.

The process of being 'prodded' and examined during pregnancy was deemed by mothers to intensify as pregnancy progressed, with mothers becoming complicit first in abdominal examinations and then with more physical and invasive procedures. Once mothers considered an examination as routine or necessary to ensure the health and well-being of their baby, they legitimised their compliance with it.

> I think I got so used to being prodded, you just get used to it . . . it is one of those things that you have to accept when you have your checks on a regular basis. You just have to get used to it.

The repetitive nature of examinations meant mothers relinquished control of access to their bodies during procedures, accepting this as the monitoring procedure associated with pregnancy, stating that it no longer 'bothered me' or that they 'didn't care'.

It is the sense of control over personal circumstances and interactions that is central to maintaining a sense of ownership over one's body (McHale and Gallagher, 2003) that is necessary for privacy maintenance. Where mothers retain a sense of ownership of, and control over, their body, they are able to deal with repetitive examinations and bodily exposure while perceiving their dignity to be intact. A decrease in the level of inhibition, linked to an increase in embarrassment of the examination, enabled mothers to temporarily transfer ownership of their privacy to the midwife in order to maintain their dignity. Midwives were then able to legitimately perform tasks on mothers' bodies without mothers challenging the need for explanations. The following mother explained:

> I don't think that it is explained enough what they are doing and why they are doing it and why it is necessary. It was just a case of right here we go, and you just lay back without any sense of explanation really.

Mothers described how a lack of explanations prior to what were considered routine procedures resulted in depersonalisation, a decline in interactions with professionals and a perceived reduction in staff's need to show them respect. Mothers in return felt unable to ask questions because of their lack of understanding of what was happening and their embarrassment caused by the processes involved. This is particularly relevant for healthcare practitioners, as guidance on informed consent prior to all procedures is explicit within professional guidance documentation (Berg *et al*, 2001; Aveyard, 2002; Royal College of Nursing, 2005). Where explanations were not given, mothers felt midwives were disrespectful and breached their privacy and dignity. This lack of respect resulted in mothers constructing strategies for dealing with invasive procedures by psychologically withdrawing from the situation in order to preserve their dignity.

Now consider Reflective activity 8.1.

Reflective activity 8.1

Consider your own area of practice and how invasive or embarrassing procedures are explained to patients:

➤ do patients ask questions about procedures that could be perceived as embarrassing?
➤ how are these procedures explained?

SOLITUDE AND WITHDRAWAL: A DIGNITY PROTECTION

Withdrawal from social interaction is portrayed within classic privacy literature as synonymous with social isolation, or being separated from a group
and free from observation (Westin, 1970; Simmel, 1971). The need for withdrawal or solitude is portrayed as necessary to our everyday lives and necessary to enhance our freedom to define ourselves (Fried, 1970; Rossler, 2005).
It is required to enable us to 'break from role-playing and the opportunity
for "making fools of ourselves"' (Rossler, 2005, p.149) and needed for 'deso-
cialisation' from others (Halmos, 1953). During pregnancy and childbirth,
withdrawal is identified by two concepts. Firstly, women may withdraw from
social interaction, as an attempt to psychologically escape from overcrowded
rooms, being viewed while breastfeeding, or reducing interactions with people
with whom mothers are not acquainted. In these instances mothers perceived
themselves as having little control over their privacy maintenance, with a subsequent result of a loss of privacy and dignity that was outside their control.
Secondly, mothers use withdrawal positively as a method of dealing with pain
during labour or examinations, which I have labelled self-introversion, that is,
withdrawing psychologically into their bodies with the aim of concentrating
on pain management. This withdrawal or self-introversion is a subconscious
adaptation process adopted by mothers as a means of securing personal privacy and a sense of control over their dignity and personal respect. Now consider Reflective activity 8.2.

Reflective activity 8.2

Most hospital wards consist of multi-occupancy rooms. Think what it must
be like to be in one of these rooms:

➤ what would you like and dislike about sharing a room with other
people?
➤ how would you feel if invasive procedures took place in this
environment?

Self-introversion

Self-introversion is a coping mechanism adopted by mothers while concentrating on managing the physical side of labour. It enables mothers to ignore social
events, social interactions and the discourse surrounding them. For most individuals, isolation, under normal circumstances, is a function associated with
defining and redefining ourselves. Its function is to enhance personal autonomy, aid emotional release and promote self-evaluation while limiting and
protecting interactions and communication with others, all of which are per-

ceived as necessary for daily living (Westin, 1970; Rossler, 2005). The process of daily living requires us to 'act a part' within society or, as Goffman (1959) states, the 'belief in the part one is playing'. By utilising self-introversion, mothers are able to suspend the role they usually play as partner, wife or mother and concentrate on the process of childbirth. This allows them to act differently from the norm during labour, without any associated embarrassment. For example, mothers in labour may remove all clothing without being inhibited by their nakedness, and upon reflection they promote this as a normal action.

By psychologically separating the body from the pain, such as that caused by labour or invasive physical examinations, the experience becomes something that happens physically *to your body* and not personally *to you*. Bodily detachment or disassociation from the body enables mothers to disassociate themselves from procedures, what Rachels (1975) describes as 'property rights', as a coping mechanism and to reduce any later embarrassment. By temporarily disassociating from the body, mothers subconsciously enable others to claim ownership of it, with subsequent right of possession and legitimate access. While Rachels perceived this disownership of the body as detrimental and disempowering within nursing, within midwifery, ownership is temporarily transferred by the mother voluntarily to the midwife. As temporary ownership is re-established to the midwife, she becomes the new *'owner'*, with right of access to the mother's body, enabling her to act on her behalf and address her privacy needs without consent, what Lawler (1991) calls 'an environment of permission'. As witnessed during participant observation, mothers handed over control of addressing privacy requirements to the midwife, so that when people knocked on doors or accessed rooms mothers no longer needed to pull down their clothing, cover themselves, or even acknowledge that person, leaving these superficial tasks to their midwife. This reallocation of basic privacy management was not verbally acknowledged between mothers and midwife, but undertaken through a subconscious awareness of each other, focused upon the individual needs of the mother.

It is important to note that self-introversion only takes place in the presence of a distraction, such as pain. Where a mother finds herself in a situation where pain is removed, such as when an epidural is used or where she has an operative delivery under spinal anaesthesia, then the need for introversion is decreased. In instances such as these, mothers' senses increase as they listen to and observe what is happening around them.

Now read through Box 8.1 and consider how Jessica might have felt in this situation.

When visiting Jessica in the postnatal period, we discussed her birthing experience, and in particular her experience at and following the birth. She described her sense of shame and embarrassment at being exposed like a 'slab of meat' for all to see, and of her 'horror' of events. She clearly remembered

---

BOX 8.1 *Jessica's story*

During a participant observation I shadowed an experienced midwife in the operating theatre when a mother arrived for an emergency birth. The birth progressed quickly under spinal anaesthesia and the baby was born in good condition. At the end of the operation the mother was observed lying naked on the table with her gown around her neck. Her body was completely exposed and no-one took the time to cover her. In the room was her partner, the anaesthetist, an operating theatre technician, a midwife, a student midwife and a healthcare assistant. It wasn't until the senior midwife returned that the mother was covered and her sanitary towels reapplied and someone spoke to her. Throughout the observation the door to the operating theatre was open and visitors could be seen walking along the adjoining corridor.

---

people talking in the theatre and walking by in the corridor. For example, she told me all about the social life of two members of staff as they described what they would be doing at the weekend. Jessica also described two activities experienced just before and just after the birth. She outlined how before the birth, once her pain was removed through spinal anaesthesia, she became more aware of those around her. She described how she listened to every word, fearing for the safety of her baby, watching everything that everyone was doing. She feared that there was a problem with her baby and ended up lying completely still and non-participative in order not to distract the professionals from their work, for fear of hindering their attempts to deliver her child. Once the birth was completed, this heightened awareness of senses remained, but at this stage she knew that her baby was safe and removed to the care of her partner. She then focused on what was occurring around her. She found herself looking at her naked body lying on the operating table. No-one appeared to be concerned for her dignity or respected the need for her body to be covered. Staff started to tidy up and move items around the room; the operating theatre doors were opened, exposing her to visitors walking along the corridor. She felt very alone and disrespected and at this stage she cried:

> . . . the whole time I was like "Oh my god" what have they seen? That was quite important to me but of course at the time you don't care too much but you still do, it is still your dignity.

Staff deal with mothers in the operating theatre as if they are unconscious patients, forgetting that the majority have spinal anaesthesia and are awake throughout the process. By ignoring their privacy needs and showing a lack of respect for mothers' bodily needs, mothers perceive themselves as no more than slabs of meat on the table. In contrast, midwives within the privacy study stated that one of their key roles was to protect the privacy and dignity of mothers by acting as advocate for them in situations where they perceived the mothers to be compromised. This appeared to be the case in situations where mothers laboured in individual rooms, under the auspices of a single midwife, but was not the case where the pregnancy became compromised.

In situations of compromise mothers perceived themselves to be watched by others, and ignored during conversations between practitioners. This resulted in mothers perceiving care as something that is 'done to them' rather than a mutual participation between parties. Subsequently, mothers experience a loss of ownership of their body which increased their sense of vulnerability and exposed them to increased physical contact by healthcare professionals, all of which were compounded by the attitudes of hospital staff, which mothers perceived to be patronising and authoritarian. In a study by Applegate and Morse (1994), where care home residents were viewed as objects, privacy needs were violated and patients became invisible or dehumanised, with privacy considered unnecessary or unimportant. Being treated as an object is not always initiated or perpetuated by staff. Within my study, mothers also adopted the role of inanimate object in order not to influence the work of doctors and midwives, when the safety of their baby was perceived to be compromised. Adopting this role was sensed as positive by mothers – as something they had to do short-term, was requirement specific, and necessary to achieve their primary goal of a healthy baby and safe return home.

In contrast, mothers admitted into single rooms on delivery suites, when in established labour, are more likely to achieve physical control of their privacy through isolation from the rest of society, by staking a claim on their room and having their birthing partner present. If mothers felt safe and secure in their environment, and with their midwife, they expressed some control over associated events. This sense of control over their labour ensured that as pain levels increased they were able to achieve privacy and maintain a sense of dignity by managing their pain through self-introversion. Where mothers felt in control of their labour pain they were able to concentrate on their body and their breathing, resulting in them becoming desensitised to surrounding events, for example:

> . . . you are in a bubble. You are in your own world and as far as I was concerned it was just me and my husband.

> Partner: I think during the delivery Rose wouldn't have noticed if there had been a coach full of Japanese tourists come through quite frankly [laughter].
> Rose: No, I can't remember half the things that I went through.

Goffman (1961, p.61) describes this type of situational withdrawal as 'regression' or 'plateaux of disinvolvement', where the person withdraws their attention from everything apart from what is happening in their immediate vicinity, and views these events in a different way than other people present do. This withdrawal enables mothers to remain in a 'birthing reality', which is then exited at the point of the birth. This enables mothers to disassociate themselves from the pain and in some cases the indignity of childbirth, in order for them to progress into their new role as a mother.

THE INDIGNITY OF WARD-BASED TREATMENT

In a number of cases, mothers are admitted to hospital in early labour. These mothers do not remain on the delivery suite but are transferred to the antenatal ward until labour is established. During this admission mothers are cared for within 4–6-bedded rooms, having all of their treatments and examinations undertaken within this public environment. Treatments and examinations undertaken include insertion of vaginal pessaries, vaginal examinations and daily examinations of abdomen and vaginal loss. While these treatments are not usually problematic if undertaken in the right environment, they become problematic when completed in the public environment of the ward. It is human nature that visitors and other mothers like to eavesdrop on conversations in the wards, as we all like a good gossip and the drama of unusual events. In the ward environment, mothers envisage eavesdroppers visualising invasive procedures taking place behind the curtains and confirmed that they too listened to conversations between mother and midwife. The following mothers described their experiences:

> This person just arrived and said "right I am going to put this pessary in" and nobody told you how awful this was going to be, on the ward there was just like a thin curtain around you and like other women on the ward as well and it was horrible.

> I think it depends where you are because I was in the ward with six other women that was fine when they were coming round giving you treatments but they were quite painful and some of them were due in visiting times when men were there and all you have got is a very thin curtain and some treatments that are quite intimate. You know, they are being described to you exactly what is going to happen and what you are going to feel and then they are pushing and shoving and what have you, and you are reacting to this, or are going to and on the other side of the very thin curtain you know, is a lady with her family and her husband and what have you. I found that most embarrassing.

Induction of labour and the insertion of vaginal pessaries caused most concern for mothers in relation to embarrassment caused by a loss of privacy and dignity during examinations. They were concerned that they might scream and embarrass themselves and others. There was a perception that staff perceived the curtains to provide enough privacy for them and, although this may be the case with protection from visual privacy, this was counterproductive when midwives described in detail the process of examinations. One mother stated: 'you are private but you are not, you can hear everything'.

The outcomes of procedures in the ward were embarrassment, a loss of dignity for mothers and a sense of loss of control over personal details and intimate aspects of care. The embarrassment caused to mothers was enhanced by the silent acknowledgement of the experience by others present in the room. As the curtains were drawn back each person in the room had some idea of what had occurred, yet there was no acknowledgement of such and so mothers remained embarrassed. One mother, when discussing the implications of her care in the ward, said 'I hate to think about it'. In response to discussions on improving privacy in the ward mothers in the study suggested the use of a 'treatment room' where they could go for treatment, 'just you and the midwife', without the fear of being overlooked or overheard by others.

Now carry out Reflective activity 8.3.

Reflective activity 8.3

How do you think privacy and dignity could be achieved in a ward environment? Consider both the environment and staff behaviour in your response.

LOSS OF FACE: BEING OVERHEARD WHILE IN LABOUR

Mothers who find themselves on an antenatal ward when in early labour describe themselves as 'performing' in front of others. Their need to act instinctively in labour is hindered by the number of people in the environment and mothers' feelings of being in a public setting. They describe themselves as wanting to be able to be themselves and act as they wanted by 'screaming out' or 'moaning', but felt restricted in the presence of others. This is because mothers are acutely aware of the impact their actions have on other occupants and describe themselves as not wanting to lose face in front of others. This loss of face is described as not being able to cope with pain or of making a fool of yourself, which is in turn perceived by them to reflect their failure as a mother. Where mothers deemed themselves unable to cope with examinations or being overheard by others, this resulted in a sense of shame and loss of face (Goffman, 1959, 1963; Rykwert, 2001). These feelings were compounded by the perception that midwives 'aren't bothered' about the mothers' privacy and have no respect for them or their pain or discomfort. One mother stated:

> It [privacy] is of absolutely no importance to the staff there at all. Because you are on the production line, in fairness to them, they are racing around like people possessed, there is hardly any staff and there are far too many people and they have to try and get on with the job in hand and unfortunately as quickly as possible.

The mothers' perception of being on a 'production line' does nothing to enhance self-worth or empowerment, and results in feelings of stupidity, uselessness, vulnerability and disempowerment. As staff were perceived as too busy, privacy became compromised and care became something that was 'done to you' without regard to privacy needs, and completed in a busy and overcrowded environment. Once mothers' private 'face' became public, personal information about them moved into the public sphere, to include the way they behaved and their personal and intimate details, all of which were perceived as an invasion of personal privacy and a loss of personal dignity.

The notion of labouring in front of other people makes mothers feel they are on display and having their ability to cope examined by others. Prospective mothers described how during labour they were going to remain mobile, dressed and maintain a sense of dignity throughout. In reality they found themselves in a public environment, on display and in fear of impending events due to the observation of others. The onset of labour is associated with onset of pain, however minor. Often, as seen during participant observation, mothers laboured in wards behind closed curtains resulting in other mothers overhearing them during labour without witnessing the event. This can be linked to the experience of visiting the dentist, where the dental drill is heard and the level of perceived pain we are going to experience enhanced, even before we have entered the surgery. Overhearing another mother's pain was deemed to be an extensive privacy breach at what mothers perceived to be a private time.

> There were people in the early stages of labour in beds around this ward with only a curtain around them, who were clearly in pain, there were people moaning and so on and I thought "I can't face this" . . . I thought that there was no privacy for me.

> There were all these women, I think it was busy downstairs [on the delivery suite] and they would be walking up and down, moaning in pain and waiting to go down and we would have paid the midwives not to hear that.

Mothers perceived that the idea that you are being watched or overheard when in labour, reflected on their ability to remain unseen or unheard at this very private time. They did not want to feel compromised by the views or attitudes of others and did not want to feel that they were making a fool of themselves in public.

Mothers' perceptions were that once pain commenced they should be transferred to a single room on the delivery suite. In retrospect mothers felt they were kept on wards far too long and in so doing were deprived of the privacy of a single room. Mothers determined that if labour progressed to the point where they were in pain, then they should be 'allowed to go on to the delivery suite' and that decision should be theirs and not the practitioner's, the rationale being:

> when your labour does start, you need to be taken somewhere even if it is not delivery suite because they can't take you [on delivery suite] but a side room, where you are not worried about screaming in front of a lot of people.

Overhearing mothers in pain was not the only perceived breach of privacy and dignity. As the ward environments are spatially challenged, the possibility of other people overhearing conversations involving personal aspects of your life or pregnancy is significantly increased; this was the case with Lindsey (see Box 8.2).

BOX 8.2 *Lindsey's story*

Lindsey had been admitted to the accident and emergency department following the onset of acute abdominal pain. She subsequently delivered a healthy baby boy. Lindsey had a concealed pregnancy, stating that she was not aware that she was pregnant. After the birth she was admitted to a six-bedded postnatal ward. The midwife ensured Lindsey was placed in bed and then brought a portable telephone so that she could contact her mother. She telephoned her mother to explain her situation and asked for her to visit. Her mother commenced an in-depth conversation on what had happened and Lindsey found herself discussing her experience in detail in front of the other mothers in the ward.

On discussion with other mothers in the ward they told me in graphic terms about Lindsey's experience, describing in detail issues relating to her pregnancy, labour and shock at being a new mother. The indignity of being placed in this situation was overwhelming for Lindsey. The whole process of ensuring that you maintain your dignity during pregnancy and childbirth focuses upon the respect that a mother has for herself and her situation. By placing mothers, in this case Lindsey, in a position where their private life is under scrutiny, in what is a sensitive situation, a person's ability to ensure their own privacy and maintain their self-respect is decreased. While this example could be considered extreme, it can be applied to similar situations, for example where healthcare professionals discuss cases behind curtains or in a public place while the mother or patient is present. Now carry out Reflective activity 8.4, based on Lindsey's story.

Reflective activity 8.4

➤ Reflect upon Lindsey's predicament and consider how a practitioner could have helped her maintain her self-respect and dignity in this situation.

➤ Consider your own practice environment and reflect upon any similar situations that may have occurred and how they can be prevented.

CONCLUSION

Privacy and dignity are interrelated concepts. Without privacy a mother has no protective mechanism to maintain her dignity. The repetitive nature of examinations during pregnancy and birth desensitises mothers to their invasive nature. This helps mothers determine what is necessary for monitoring the health of their baby so they are considered as part of the normal childbearing process. By achieving this status, a mother does not perceive her dignity to be compromised. In situations where mothers are participating in a normal birth, then it is important for the midwife to act as advocate for the mother to ensure that her privacy and dignity needs continue to be met while the mother engages in self-introversion. However, where a mother finds herself in a situation of compromise, such as when admitted to an antenatal ward or requiring an operative delivery, it is important for healthcare professionals to ensure that mothers are treated with respect. Where mothers feel they are not respected and their privacy is not promoted, then they perceive their dignity to be compromised after their baby is born. Healthcare professionals have a role to play in ensuring that mothers maintain their dignity during pregnancy and childbirth, to ensure they have a positive birthing experience.

REFERENCES

Applegate M, Morse J (1994) Personal privacy and interactional patterns in a nursing home. *Journal of Ageing Studies* **8**(4): 413–34.

Aveyard H (2002) The requirement for informed consent prior to nursing care procedures. *Journal of Advanced Nursing* **37**(3): 243–9.

Berg J, Appelbaum P, Lidz C, Parker L (2001) *Informed Consent: legal theory and clinical practice* (2e). New York: Oxford University Press Inc.

Bloustein E (2003) *Individual and Group Privacy.* London: Transaction Publishers.

Burden B (2007) *Privacy in Maternity Care Environments.* Unpublished PhD thesis. Buckingham: Open University.

Fried C (1970) *An Anatomy of Values.* Cambridge, MA: Harvard University Press.

Goffman E (1959) *The Presentation of Self in Everyday Life.* London: Penguin Books.

Goffman E (1961) *Asylums: essays on the social situation of mental patients and other inmates.* New York: Doubleday.

Goffman E (1963) *Behavior in Public Places.* New York: The Free Press.

Goffman E (1967) *Interaction Ritual: essays on face-to-face behavior.* New York: Pantheon Books.

Halmos P (1953) *Solitude and Privacy: a study of social isolation, its causes and therapy.* New York: Philosophical Library Inc.

Lawler J (1991) *Behind the Screens: nursing somology and the problem of the body.* London: Churchill Livingstone.

McHale J, Gallagher A (2003) *Nursing and Human Rights.* London: Butterworth Heinemann.

Rachels J (1975) Why privacy is important. *Philosophy and Public Affairs* 4: 323–33.

Rosen J (2001) *The Unwanted Gaze: the destruction of privacy in America.* New York: Vintage.

Rossler B (2005) *The Value of Privacy.* Cambridge: Polity Press.

Royal College of Nursing (2005) *Informed Consent in Health and Social Care Research: RCN guidance for nurses.* London: Royal College of Nursing.

Rykwert J (2001) Privacy in antiquity. *Social Research* 68(1): 29–40.

Schneider C (1977) *Shame, Exposure and Privacy.* London: WW Norton and Company.

Simmel A (1971) Privacy is not an isolated freedom. In: Pennock, JR, Chapman JW (eds) *Privacy.* New York: Atherton.

Westin A (1970) *Privacy and Freedom.* London: The Bodley Head.

CHAPTER 9

Dignity and older people

Wilfred McSherry and Helen Coleman

INTRODUCTION

Statistics tell us that currently within the United Kingdom (UK) and globally, there are more people aged 80 years and over than those aged 16 years and below (Office for National Statistics, 2010). We don't have to be mathematicians to predict that at some point in the future this will have a significant impact on all sections of our society but especially with regard to those working within the health and social care sectors.

Ageing is non-discriminatory, it comes to all people because it is a natural and inevitable process as one moves along the life span continuum from birth to death. However, in contemporary society, ageing seems to be feared and discussions on the subject avoided. Until the advent of an 'elixir of life' or the development of genetic engineering that switches off or halts the ageing process, everyone is destined to grow old – unless they die prematurely. Therefore, the fact that we are all destined to live longer, fuller and healthier lives should be a cause for celebration, and the contribution that older people make to the fabric, culture and social structure of society remembered and welcomed. For some older people, retirement or social ageing is positive, enjoyable and life enhancing. It is an opportunity to spend time with family and friends, participating in recreational activities, engaging in new pursuits and experiences. However, for others ageing will mean a decline in physical and cognitive functioning as a result of illness, disease or trauma. This may result in increased morbidity, a loss of independence and social isolation. The onset of illness or disease may result in periods of hospitalisation. Depending on the nature and severity of an illness or disease, this may necessitate long-term health and social care. The quality of this care has the potential to preserve the older person's dignity and identity or rob them of a fundamental aspect of their humanity and human rights.

Health and social care professionals are in a unique and privileged position to safeguard and preserve the dignity of older people. Therefore, this chapter will first explore why dignity is important for older people and why older people might be vulnerable to a loss of dignity, drawing on research findings and reports about older people's dignity. The chapter will explain what is important for older people's dignity, by providing illustrated examples of where dignified care for older people may not have been achieved in various settings.

LEARNING OUTCOMES

By the end of this chapter you will be able to:
➤ understand what is meant by the phrase 'dignity in care' when caring for older people
➤ demonstrate an awareness of how care and services may be organised to preserve the dignity of older people
➤ be aware of the strategies that can safeguard the dignity of older people
➤ transfer the knowledge and skills gained throughout this chapter into the delivery of health and social care.

DEMOGRAPHICS OF AGEING

The World Health Organization (2000) estimates that by 2025, there will be 1.2 billion people in the world over the age of 60 years. In developing countries the over-60s will account for 70% of the populations. Interestingly, the fastest-growing age group is the over-80s.

These statistics suggest that globally the number of older people is due to increase. The fact that more people are living longer in the developed and developing world should not really be viewed negatively, but should be a cause for celebration. There have been tremendous improvements in health, education and welfare, eradicating diseases and illness. Changes in welfare standards such as sanitation and housing, and measures taken to remove poverty and social inequality have all contributed to an increased life expectancy.

It is easy to look at statistics and figures and think that these do not really matter because they are not directly relevant. The following may help to illustrate how these global trends in relation to older people directly impact upon healthcare.

➤ We undertook a review of the patients who were in hospital on one day. Over 68% of all the people in hospital were over the age of 65 years, with a large proportion being over the age of 80 years.

This finding illustrates that the global predictions with regard to an increasing older population are occurring within the UK. They also indicate why there is a need to look at dignity and older people, because older people are the largest consumers of health and social care and one of the largest groups within society.

ATTITUDES TOWARD AGEING AND OLDER PEOPLE

Within some sections of society there seems to be a general lack of tolerance, sensitivity and disregard towards the needs of older people. Older people are often portrayed as a burden and demanding; healthcare is not immune to these negativities. There are many prejudices and myths that require dispelling, with regard to caring for older people (see Box 9.1).

BOX 9.1 *Reflection: dispelling myths!*

Caring for older people, especially within the acute hospital environment, suggests images of hard graft and dirty work! Not too long ago one of the authors of this chapter was dissuaded by a senior manager from applying for a nursing post within older people services. Suffice it to say that the person concerned did not listen and spent many satisfying and rewarding years caring for older people. In fact, this person learned more about care, caring, dignity and respect than they had at any other time in their nursing career. This anecdote illustrates that it is not all doom and gloom and detrimental to one's nursing career, as implied by the senior manager; on the contrary, nursing older people is professionally fulfilling and enabling.

The above reflection emphasises the need for us all to challenge our attitudes towards ageing. The so-called age or generation gap still exists, despite many drives in society and health and social care to eradicate age discrimination and stereotyping in the drive for equality (Department of Health [DH], 2001). The fact that there is a chapter in this book dedicated to dignity and the older person is itself a form of discrimination. It highlights that the needs and perceptions of older people are different from those of other groups within society. However, this form of discrimination is positive because it focuses attention on how older people may perceive dignity and respect and how intergenerational differences may be overcome so that their dignity and respect can be preserved, enabling older people to feel valued and integrated within society.

There are numerous incidents highlighted in the media where older people are subjected to all forms of abuse, whether emotional, physical, financial, sexual or social. Furthermore, some older people become fearful of crime, meaning they may withdraw from wider society. Evidence suggests that some older people, for example those suffering from dementia, can be treated with a general disregard and a lack of respect within our communities and within diverse healthcare settings (Alzheimer's Society, 2009). Older people can often be left feeling useless and unwanted in a society that seems to value youthfulness and beauty over wisdom, experience and knowledge. There needs to be a realisation that older people make a significant contribution to society. How many of us have relied upon grandparents to provide child care? And are we aware of the vast amount of voluntary work undertaken by older people?

Now carry out Reflective activity 9.1.

Reflective activity 9.1

Before proceeding you might want to make a note or recall some of the words, phrases or terms used to describe older people

---

Your reflections may have seen you producing a list of terms, some of which may view older people in a very negative light – terms such as 'wrinklies', 'old dear', 'old boy', 'old girl', 'pet', 'love', 'dear'. Older people are often seen as being slow, forgetful, out of touch, technophobes, unable to make decisions. While some of these stereotypical images and terms may not be intentional, they often leave older people feeling patronised, disempowered and degraded, losing self-respect and value as a person.

A sense of proportion

It would be very wrong to think that all older people are treated with a general lack of dignity and respect within society. On the contrary, for example within healthcare, many older people using healthcare services report a high level of satisfaction with the treatment and care that they receive. Garratt, for the Acute Co-ordination Centre for the NHS Patient Survey Programme (Garratt, 2009; p.2), reported that:

> Nearly 8 in 10 patients (79%) rated the care they received in hospital as 'excellent' (43%) or 'very good' (35%) with those rating their overall care as 'excellent' increasing from 42% in 2007 to 43% in 2008 (reproduced with permission from the Picker Institute Europe).

Therefore, the vast majority of adults and older people are satisfied with the hospital care received. The challenge for all working in health and social care is to improve services for the small proportions of patients who are dissatisfied with the care provided, so that everyone is satisfied.

Dignity and older Europeans

The European Commission (2004) funded a project called Dignity and Older Europeans. This is an influential study that explored older Europeans' understanding of the concept of dignity. The project brought together academics, clinicians and user groups. Please look at the following web link for further information and access to the reports and resources that were produced: http://medic.cardiff.ac.uk/archive_subsites/_/_/medic/subsites/dignity/index.html

The findings from this study provide an in-depth account of what older people from across Europe feel about dignity, detailing how healthcare professionals can preserve the older person's dignity. Within the educational material produced it is evident that using inappropriate terms of endearment is something that many older people find intolerable, unacceptable and offensive:

➤ when meeting an older person for the first time, always call them by their family/surname, not their first name, until they have given you permission to do so. Never use inappropriate terms of endearment

➤ when caring for older people in whatever setting, always knock on the door or seek permission prior to entering their house, room or personal space.

RECENT POLICY AND PUBLICITY

Within the UK there have been a number of drives to enhance the care of older people. There are clear steps being taken across health and social care (full health economy) to raise the quality and standards of care delivered. There is a notable emphasis placed on the concepts of dignity and respect. Lord Darzi's review states:

> Quality of care includes quality of *caring*. This means how personal care is – the compassion, dignity and respect with which patients are treated. It can only be improved by analysing and understanding patient satisfaction with their own experiences (DH, 2008, p.47).

Yet, despite a great deal of investment and publicity with campaigns (DH, 2006a; Royal College of Nursing [RCN], 2008) and dignity champion programmes (DH, 2009b) seeking to raise the standards of care for all, especially older people, there are a growing number of publications emerging that highlight that older people are still being subjected to and are vulnerable to undignified care. This is despite all the drives to combat the negativities and discrepancies in care provided to older people, especially within acute care (DH, 2001).

Rayner, president of the Patients Association, writes in the foreword of the report:

> For far too long now, the Patients Association has been receiving calls on our Helpline from people wanting to talk about the dreadful, neglectful, demeaning, painful and sometimes downright cruel treatment their elderly relatives had experienced at the hands of NHS nurses (Rayner, 2009, p.3, reproduced with permission from the Patients Association).

The content of this foreword is extremely sad and concerning because it indicates that some older people are still not receiving a quality and level of care that respects their humanity, despite all the policy and guidelines attempting to reverse these negative cultural trends.

This quotation also reinforces why there is an urgent need to focus upon the dignity of older people within society and healthcare specifically.

THE MEANING OF DIGNITY FOR OLDER PEOPLE

Fenton and Mitchell (2002) provide a useful definition of dignity that underlines the fundamental principles of dignity and older people. It describes clearly what older people consider dignity to be (*see* Reflective activity 9.2).

Reflective activity 9.2

Please revisit the following definition that was referred to in Chapter 2, identifying the main dimensions of dignity, reflecting on how these may relate to older people.

> Dignity is a state of physical, emotional and spiritual comfort, with each individual valued for his or her uniqueness and his or her individuality celebrated. Dignity is promoted when individuals are enabled to do the best within their capabilities, exercise control, make choices and feel involved in the decision-making that underpins their care (Fenton and Mitchell, 2002, p.2, reproduced with permission from the RCN).

Your reflections may have revealed that older people want to be:
➤ treated in an individual and holistic manner, with equal attention paid to the physical, psychological, social and spiritual aspects of their lives
➤ accepted as unique individuals and have this individuality celebrated
➤ involved to the best of their ability in decisions and choices
➤ in control and exercise control of their own lives.

Crucially, this definition implies that dignity is fundamental to the older person's identify, self-worth and ultimately their individuality and humanity. Implicit in the word dignity is the word respect. Fenton and Mitchell's (2002) definition implies that respect concerns seeing the older person as an individual with a past, present and a future. It is all too easy to focus upon the person as a condition rather than the individual.

A theoretical model of dignity

Nordenfelt and Edgar (2005) present a theoretical model of dignity created within the Dignity and Older Europeans project. By analysing older people's responses, descriptions and experience of dignity, they were able to develop a theoretical model (Figure 9.1). This model suggests that older people described or felt that there are four types of *'dignity'*. The dashed lines indicate that all types of dignity are interrelated and share equal importance. They build on Fenton and Mitchell's (2002) definition by presenting a model that may assist healthcare professionals to understand the relevance and importance attached to dignity by older people.

Now carry out Reflective activity 9.3.

Reflective activity 9.3

Study the four types of dignity and ask yourself: what do these mean? Can you think of any examples that may illustrate these meanings within everyday life and practice?

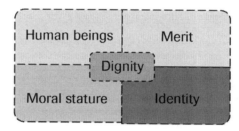

Figure 9.1 A theoretical model of dignity (Nordenfelt and Edgar, 2005).

Chapter 2 explored meanings of dignity, including Nordenfelt and Edgar's (2005) theory. Here, the four types of dignity are defined and there is application to older people.

➤ *Menschenwürde*: this word is translated from German as 'humanness'. Therefore, this type of dignity refers to the dignity inherent within every human being. This type affirms that dignity is something universal. This may indicate that dignity is now enshrined within the Human Rights Act (Great Britain, 1998) and legislation. Therefore, if we deny older people the right to express individuality and their humanity, whether intentionally or unintentionally, then we may be violating their primary right to dignity.

➤ *Dignity as merit*, either formal or informal, is dignity conferred upon someone as a result of either merit or rank. Some people may inherit titles. However, in this classification, dignity is usually earned or conferred by others because of deeds or actions. As an example of people who may be conferred a level of merit, think of a good ward manager who inspires through their leadership. Such people are conferred a level of merit from all with whom they work.

➤ *The dignity of moral stature* refers to one's own moral identity and stature and how a person may lose this if they fail to act in accordance with their guiding principles and values. Think of the recent UK scandal about 'MPs' expenses' and how the lack of moral principles displayed by some MPs shattered public trust and confidence.

➤ *The dignity of personal identity* concerns the identity of the person. A person can be robbed or violated by physical assault or humiliation. The notions of integrity and physical identity, autonomy and inclusion are all important aspects of the person's identity. This type of dignity has the most profound impact upon health and social care. If one studies this definition, it is easy to see how a healthcare professional's actions, attitudes and behaviour can either preserve a patient's identity or destroy it. This can be illustrated in the following example taken from the Healthcare Commission (2009, p.6):

> The care of patients was unacceptable. For example, patients and relatives told us that when patients rang the call bell because they were in pain or needed to go to the toilet, it was often not answered . . . Some relatives claimed that patients were left, sometimes for hours, in wet or soiled sheets . . . (Healthcare Commission, 2009, p.6, © Care Quality Commission).

It is clear that such practices had a demeaning and distressing impact upon the individual's sense of identity. These behaviours and practices robbed the individual and their families of dignity and humanity.

Now carry out Reflective activity 9.4.

Reflective activity 9.4

Spend a few minutes reading through the extract from the report. Ask yourself how would you expect to be treated?

WHAT OLDER PEOPLE WANT

The previous section highlighted some very serious failings in the care of older people. By reflecting on the implications of such reports and by assessing our own perceptions, attitudes and practices towards dignity in care, the culture within healthcare may be changed. The danger is that such reports are so painful and distressing to read that we avoid engaging with them. Yet, explicit within such reports are the foundations and recommendations for a sustained change in practice. They also tell us something about older people's expectations and standards with regard to dignity and respect.

Now carry out Reflective activity 9.5.

Reflective activity 9.5

Look at Box 9.2, which contains the DH (2006c) ten-point dignity challenge (also discussed in relation to health policy in Chapter 4). Take each clause in turn and ask yourself what this may mean for you personally and for the older people for whom you care.

BOX 9.2 *The Department of Health ten-point dignity challenge*

High-quality care services that respect people's dignity should:

1. have a zero tolerance of all forms of abuse
2. support people with the same respect you would want for yourself or a member of your family
3. treat each person as an individual by offering a personalised service
4. enable people to maintain the maximum possible level of independence, choice and control
5. listen and support people to express their needs and wants
6. respect people's right to privacy
7. ensure people feel able to complain without fear of retribution
8. engage with family members and carers as care partners
9. assist people to maintain confidence and a positive self-esteem
10. act to alleviate people's loneliness and isolation.

(Department of Health, 2006c, Crown copyright; reproduced with permission from the Controller of HMSO and the Queen's Printer for Scotland)

The origin of the DH's Dignity in Care campaign was discussed in Chapter 4. This section demonstrates how the DH (2006a,b,c) dignity challenge was introduced to raise awareness of the importance of preserving the dignity of older people. This also coincided with the recruitment of regional dignity champions who were asked to register with the DH in order to challenge some of the practices that were detrimental to older people. A full summary of the impact of dignity champions was published (DH, 2009a). A similar campaign was launched by the RCN (2008). It is sometimes easy to be cynical and think that such campaigns have little impact. However, it must be emphasised that both these campaigns have had a significant impact with regard to raising awareness of dignity in care by challenging practice, breaking down barriers and, importantly, changing cultures.

Different organisations have responded in diverse ways to implementing the dignity challenge within their organisational structures and processes. Some of the 'good practice stories' and 'bright ideas projects' initiated to promote and preserve the dignity of older people are outlined on the DH Dignity in Care website: www.dignityincare.org.uk.

Each point in the ten-point challenge relates to a fundamental aspect of dignity. For a more in-depth explanation and discussion on how each point applies to older people and healthcare, please look at the following material developed by the Health and Social Care Advisory Service (HASCAS) (2010) *Dignity Through Action (Older People) Resource Package*, which can be downloaded from: www.hascas.org/hascas_publications_downloads.shtml.

The dignity challenge alerts us to what is important for older people in preserving dignity. It focuses attention on areas that healthcare professionals must consider when caring for older people.

PRESERVING THE DIGNITY OF OLDER PEOPLE

Previous sections have outlined what older people understand by the concept of dignity. This section explores strategies, practices, behaviours and attitudes that will preserve the dignity of older people. The RCN's (2008, p.6) definition of dignity (Box 9.3) highlights a number of key factors and strategies that are central to the dignity of older people. It reveals that 'people, processes and places', as outlined in Chapter 2, must be considered when preserving the dignity of older people

---

Box 9.3 *Royal College of Nursing definition of dignity*

Dignity is concerned with how people feel, think and behave in relation to the worth or value of themselves and others. To treat someone with dignity is to treat them as being of worth, in a way that is respectful of them as valued individuals.

In care situations, dignity may be promoted or diminished by: the physical environment; organisational culture; the attitudes and behaviour of the nursing team and others; and the way in which care activities are carried out.

When dignity is present people feel in control, valued, confident, comfortable and able to make decisions for themselves. When dignity is absent people feel devalued, lacking control and comfort. They may lack confidence and be unable to make decisions for themselves. They may feel humiliated, embarrassed or ashamed.

Dignity applies equally to those who have capacity and to those who lack it. Everyone has equal worth as human beings and must be treated as if they are able to feel, think and behave in relation to their own worth or value.

The nursing team should, therefore, treat all people in all settings and of any health status with dignity, and dignified care should continue after death.

(RCN, 2008, p.6, used with kind permission from the Royal College of Nursing)

Now carry out Reflective activity 9.6.

Reflective activity 9.6

Read the case study in Box 9.4, which is an extract taken from a case presented in the Patients' Association report (2009). While reading through this, ask yourself the following questions:

➤ what steps could have been taken to preserve Ann's dignity?
➤ which of the four types of dignity are violated?
➤ how did people, processes and places influence this situation?

BOX 9.4 *Ann McNeill by her husband Richard McNeill*

My wife Ann McNeill died on 15 January 2008. Ann was 71 when she had to undergo a succession of major operations in the months preceding her death. She was a patient at both Barnet Hospital and Edgware Community Hospital, moving between the two. Ann had spent decades working as a nurse, she trained with Claire Rayner, and she put a lot of pride in the role of nurses as caring professionals.

Whilst I struggle to remember exact dates and details, during her time there were things that happened to my wife that I will remember forever. I feel that poor nursing care over a long period of time contributed to her death. Ann couldn't relate the attitude and actions of some of the nurses with how she had been trained to look after people.

In October 2007, following surgery at Barnet Hospital she was transferred to Edgware Community General Hospital in North London. It was supposed to be an intermediate step whilst she recovered. I was appalled at how my wife was treated by some of the staff. Her legs were raw and covered in bandages both to protect her wounds, and the fragile skin surrounding them as she had developed blisters and lesions from deep vein thrombosis and other problems. The dressings were supposed to be changed regularly, every few days, but the nurses at Edgware didn't bother. One night two nurses were hoisting her into bed and one handled her very roughly, knocking her legs. She gasped in pain and the nurse said 'Oh, we've got a drama queen here'. That description didn't match my wife in the slightest.

Later that night, the other nurse who had been more considerate and careful came and checked on Ann. There was blood on the bed sheets and her bandages from where she had been knocked. The other nurse said to the nurse who had shown such little care to Ann, 'you did this, now you clear it up'.

(Patients Association, 2009, p.31, used with kind permission from the Patients Association)

This case study illustrates how healthcare professionals' attitudes are fundamental to communicating empathy and an essential component of care and caring. The qualities that practitioners display in their interaction with older people can make a person feel respected, valued and important. However, the nurses in this situation showed no respect for Ann as an individual. Their actions, attitudes and words destroyed Ann's dignity, violating her humanity and sense of identity. Furthermore, the processes and places that were supposed to care for Ann failed in every respect.

Again there is a need for balance and proportion as it must be emphasised that the majority of nurses and healthcare professionals do a brilliant job in circumstances that are often difficult and challenging. But as indicated, these tragic cases must be reviewed so that lessons can be learnt and remedial action taken to prevent any reoccurrence.

FUNDAMENTAL ASPECTS OF DIGNITY FOR OLDER PEOPLE

Matiti *et al* (2007) outline several fundamental aspects of dignity. All these must be present if older people are to feel valued, respected and equal partners in society and care. These are all essential to preserving the identity and self-worth of older people. They are especially important to the delivery of world-class health and social care, irrespective of the context in which care is delivered:

➤ need for information
➤ communication
➤ how older people are addressed – courtesy

➤ choice and decision making
➤ respect
➤ treated with decency
➤ participation in care delivery
➤ autonomy and independence
➤ confidentiality
➤ privacy.

An additional one that we have added is: attitude.

Many of these are self-explanatory. These fundamentals are central to the delivery and implementation of the theoretical model of dignity outlined earlier. Similarly, if these are not incorporated in the caring relationship and organisational culture then older people will be left feeling vulnerable, isolated and potentially violated. Many organisations are now seeking to capture older people's experiences of care. Magee *et al* (2008) undertook a review of the different tools available to measure the level of dignity provided to older people. Some of the key areas outlined in this report are similar to those offered by Matiti *et al* (2007).

SAFEGUARDING THE DIGNITY OF OLDER PEOPLE

Figure 9.2 outlines the primary domains of dignity that are considered central to the dignity of older people (Magee *et al*, 2008). These domains are also evident in a number of other publications:

➤ hospital ward exit surveys
➤ DH (2009b) *Dignity Maps*
➤ DH (2003) *Essence of Care Patient-focused Benchmarks for Clinical Governance*
➤ Social Care Institute For Excellence (2006) *SCIE Guide 15: Dignity in Care*
➤ Magee *et al* (2008) *Measuring Dignity in Care for Older People*
➤ Healthcare Commission (2009) *Investigation into Mid Staffordshire NHS Foundation Trust*
➤ The Patients Association (2009) *Patients . . . Not Numbers, People . . . Not Statistics.*

Many organisations are now assessing these domains to determine the overall quality and standard of care provided. These areas have also been recognised by older people as being essential to preserving dignity (The Patients Association, 2009; Alzheimer's Society, 2009).

Our organisation has developed a 'Care with Dignity Indicator Tool' as one measure that can be used to capture older people's experience and satisfaction with the quality of care received. The different domains are described below. It

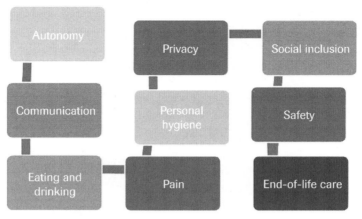

Figure 9.2 Domains of dignity (Magee *et al*, 2008).

must be emphasised that these domains are not in any order of priority since they are all essential to older people whether delivering care in a residential setting or hospital. Some of these domains are also relevant and appropriate in everyday interaction with older people.

➤ *Autonomy*: means involving the older person in decisions about their life, future and care or treatment.

➤ *Communication*: listening to and facilitating positive communication with the older person. Being non-patronising and courteous at all times.

➤ *Eating and drinking*: older people must be given control about the food they eat by offering choice. Appropriate, timely and sensitive assistance should be given with eating and drinking if this is required. Nutritional support is essential to maintain and aid recovery and the general well-being of the person.

➤ *Privacy*: the older person's privacy must be maintained and preserved at all times, especially when carrying out personal care or when using wash or toilet facilities. Consideration must be given to the location of care – whether or not this is the older person's own home. Personal space is important and older people like to feel secure and safe. Curtains must be drawn, doors closed and personal space respected. Consent should be obtained prior to carrying out any care or examinations and older people tell us that permission should be gained for students to be in attendance or for them to carry out essential care. Knocking on doors and seeking consent to enter, whether a cubicle or the person's own home, is funda-mental. All caring environments should comply with national directives regarding single-sex accommodation.

➤ *Personal hygiene*: a loss of independence and autonomy can have a very profound impact on older people's sense of worth and identity. Providing timely assistance and involving the older person in personal care empowers and removes the loss of control that can be experienced. It is imperative that older people are given a choice in decisions made about their own personal hygiene. There is a need to ensure all facilities are clean and suitable.

➤ *Pain*: there must be timely and appropriate intervention for pain or discomfort. It must be remembered that older people or their carers may know more about the treatment and management of their condition than the person providing care. This knowledge and expertise must be acknowledged and respected. The older person could be responsible for their own pain relief, should this be desired. There must be avoidance of practices that may cause or contribute to the older person experiencing pain or discomfort.

➤ *Social inclusion*: older people should be able to practise and maintain their own personal, religious and spiritual beliefs. Nurses should value the older person, ensuring that there is no age discrimination. Contact and access should be maintained with family, friends and community, if requested.

➤ *Safety*: nurses must undertake a thorough individualised assessment of each older person, identifying potential environmental or personal risks; these may include assessments for falls, use of bed rails, mobility, pressure area care, nutrition support, and necessary documentation completed. Where required, refer people to the protection of vulnerable adults team in suspected cases of elder abuse or neglect. Nursing staff must comply with all infection and prevention control measures.

➤ *End-of-life care*: death is an inevitable part of life and growing old. Older people indicate that there needs to be openness and willingness on the part of healthcare professionals to discuss and support older people with decisions that they may have made with regard to their own death. There is a danger of adopting a paternalistic attitude when dealing with matters of death and dying, to protect the older person from additional suffering. This practice must be avoided and older people must be consulted, informed and involved in all decisions made. Consideration must be given to advance directives and 'living wills'. Nurses must be culturally sensitive to religious or spiritual needs and have awareness of how these may impact upon attitudes to death and care of the person following death. Provision must be made to discuss personal wishes and preferences about end-of-life care.

CONCLUSION

This chapter has explored dignity and older people. It has highlighted what older people across Europe consider dignity to be and how dignity can be preserved within everyday interactions. It is evident that the interpersonal skills and qualities displayed and the attitudes adopted are critical when dealing with older people, whether in a caring context or in general encounters. Dealing with older people requires sensitivity and communication that is non-patronising. It must be remembered that older people are equal members of society, who have made and are still making a significant contribution to its welfare and structure. Older people must always be treated with courtesy and respect. There is a fundamental need for all of society to confront ageism, prejudice and discrimination wherever these are encountered, so that negative attitudes can be eradicated and growing old is celebrated and not feared.

REFERENCES

Alzheimer's Society (2009) *Counting the Cost Caring for People with Dementia on Hospital Wards.* London: Alzheimer's Society. http://alzheimers.org.uk/site/scripts/download_info.php?fileID=787 (accessed 11 October 2010).

Cardiff University (2004) *Dignity and Older Europeans: Final Report.* Cardiff: Cardiff University. www.cardiff.ac.uk/medic/subsites/dignity/index.html (accessed 11 October 2010).

Department of Health (2001) *National Service Framework for Older People.* London: Department of Health.

Department of Health (2003) *Essence of Care Patient-focused Benchmarks for Clinical Governance.* London: Department of Health.

Department of Health (2006a) *'Dignity in Care' Public Survey, October 2006. Report of the survey.* London: Department of Health. www.dh.gov.uk/prod_consum_dh/groups/dh_digitalassets/@dh/@en/documents/digitalasset/dh_4139558.pdf (accessed 11 October 2010).

Department of Health (2006b) *Dignity in Care. A Report on People's Views, October 2006. What you had to say. . .* London: Department of Health. www.dh.gov.uk/prod_consum_dh/groups/dh_digitalassets/@dh/@en/documents/digitalasset/dh_4139559.pdf (accessed 11 October 2010).

Department of Health (2006c) *Dignity Challenge: high quality care services that respect people's dignity.* London: Department of Health. www.dh.gov.uk/prod_consum_dh/groups/dh_digitalassets/documents/digitalasset/dh_085105.pdf (accessed 11 October 2010).

Department of Health (2008) *High Quality Care For All – NHS Next Stage Review Final report.* Gateway reference 10106. London: Department of Health.

Department of Health (2009a) *Final Report on the Department of Health's Dignity Campaign.* www.dhcarenetworks.org.uk/_library/Opinion_Leader_Final_Report_to_DH.doc.pdf (accessed 11 October 2010).

Department of Health (2009b) *Dignity Maps.* London: Department of Health. www.dhcarenetworks.org.uk/dignityincare/Topics/championresources/Dignity_Map/ (accessed 11 October 2010).

European Commission (2004) *Educating for Dignity. Dignity and older Europeans. A multi-disciplinary workbook.* http://medic.cardiff.ac.uk/archive_subsites/_/_/medic/subsites/dignity/resources/Educating_for_Dignity.pdf (accessed 11 October 2010).

Fenton E, Mitchell T (2002) Growing old with dignity: a concept analysis. *Nursing Older People* **14**(4): 19–21.

Garratt E (2009) *The Key Findings Report From the 2008 Inpatient Survey. Acute Co-ordination Centre for The NHS Patient Survey Programme 2008.* Oxford: Picker Institute Europe. www.nhssurveys.org/Filestore//documents/Key_Findings_report_for_the_2008_ Inpatient_Survey.pdf (accessed 11 October 2010).

Healthcare Commission (2009) *Investigation into Mid Staffordshire Foundation Trust.* London: Commission for Healthcare Audit and Inspection.

Human Rights Act (1998) www.opsi.gov.uk/acts/acts1998/ukpga 19980042 en 1 (accessed 11 October 2010).

Magee H, Parsons S, Askham J (2008) *Measuring Dignity in Care for Older People.* London: Picker Institute Europe for Help the Aged.

Matiti M, Cotrel-Gibbons E, Teasdale K (2007) Promoting patient dignity in healthcare settings. *Nursing Standard* **21**(45): 46–52.

Nordenfelt L, Edgar A (2005) The four notions of dignity. *Quality in Ageing* **6**(1): 17–21.

Office for National Statistics (2008) *Ageing: fastest increase in the 'oldest old'.* National Statistics. www.statistics.gov.uk/cci/nugget.asp?id=949 (accessed 11 October 2010).

Patients Association (2009) *Patients . . . Not Numbers, People . . . Not Statistics.* London: Patients Association.

Rayner C (2009) Foreword. In: *Patients . . . Not Numbers, People . . . Not Statistics.* London: Patients Association.

Royal College of Nursing (2008) *Defending Dignity – Challenges and Opportunities for Nursing.* London: Royal College of Nursing.

Social Care Institute for Excellence (2006) *SCIE Guide 15: Dignity in Care.* London: Social Care Institute for Excellence. www.scie.org.uk/publications/guides/guide15/ index.asp (accessed 11 October 2010).

World Health Organization (2000) *Social Development and Ageing: Crisis or Opportunity?* Geneva: World Health Organization. www.who.int/ageing/publications/development/ alc_social_development.pdf (accessed 11 October 2010).

CHAPTER 10

Dignity at the end of life

Davina Porock

INTRODUCTION

Dignity is one of the first things people mention when asked about the care they would like at the end of life. However, understanding what people really mean by dignity is not easy because most people have a great deal of difficulty in saying what they mean by it. In fact, mostly we know how it feels when we have lost our dignity rather than how it feels when we have dignity. Not only that, but most people do not like thinking and talking about their own death and unfortunately health professionals also find it difficult to talk to their patients about planning for end-of-life care (Hopkinson *et al*, 2003). As a result, facilitating high-quality end-of-life care that promotes dignity is sometimes very difficult to achieve.

The purpose of this chapter is to explore why dignity is so important at the end of life and how we, as health professionals, can facilitate respect for dignity with the dying person and their family. The chapter is divided into two main sections: the meaning of dignity at the end of life, and facilitating dignified dying. The chapter will focus mainly on dying and death in older age groups because that is predominantly when death occurs in our society. There are texts available on the specialist area of care of dying children and young people, for example Pfund and Fowler-Kerry (2010).

LEARNING OUTCOMES

By the end of this chapter you will be able to:
➤ describe the context of dying and death in the modern United Kingdom and consider the implications of current trends
➤ identify social and historical themes that influence our understanding of a good death and dignity at the end of life
➤ reflect on dignity, suffering and comfort as interrelated concepts that have particular meaning and resonance in care at the end of life
➤ identify practical but meaningful actions to promote dignity at the end of life.

THE MEANING OF DIGNITY AT THE END OF LIFE

There is one assured fact for any living being and that is the reality that we will die. No matter how long science can increase the length of human life with improvements in health and technology, we will still all die. We spend our lives mostly *not* thinking of this fact, and yet the threat of death is very much integrated into the way we organise our lives and respond to risk – from what we eat, to wearing a seat belt or washing our hands (Douglas, 2004). Every health professional will come in contact with dying and death even if they do not specialise in palliative care. Most people who are dying, whether it is from cancer or non-malignant disease, will be cared for by health professionals who are not palliative care specialists (Shipman *et al*, 2007). Although admissions to hospital are more frequent as patients approach death, it is unlikely that specialist palliative care teams will direct the care or even be consulted as part of the care. The last year of life is most commonly spent in the community, being cared for by family and friends with the support of district nurses, the general practitioner and community health and social services (Shipman *et al*, 2007; Gomes and Higginson, 2008).

In this section we will look first at when and where death occurs in the United Kingdom (UK), how it has changed over the past decades, and what it will look like in the future if current trends continue, as this will set the context for understanding dignity and the barriers to care provision at the end of life. Then, we will explore the research about people's preferences for end-of-life care and their concerns around dignity. The differences between what is happening and what people want, and how that affects the sense of dignity that people experience in end-of-life care, will be discussed.

DEATH: PAST, PRESENT AND FUTURE

Looking at death statistics in the UK reveals some interesting information. Table 10.1 shows the distribution of deaths over age groups in 2005 (Department of Health [DH], 2005). What can be seen from this table is that in the UK, as in all western developed countries, death is most common in older people. Over 80% of deaths occur in people over the age of 65 years, and two-thirds of all deaths occur in people over 75 years. Furthermore, two-thirds of acute hospital beds are occupied by people over 65 years of age (DH, 2005), with one-quarter of all hospital patients being people in their last year of life (Higginson *et al*, 1998). From this it can be seen that those at greatest risk of dying are old or very old and they are often in contact with acute health services in addition to community health and social services.

Currently in the UK, almost 80% of all deaths each year occur in either a hospital or a nursing home, with hospitals accounting for close to 60%. Only 19% of deaths occur at home and less than 5% of deaths occur in hospices

Table 10.1 Summary of death statistics (Office for National Statistics, 2009)

Age group (years)	Total deaths (%)
≤14	0.9
15–44	3.5
45–64	13.1
65–74	16.2
75–84	30.5
≥85	35.8

(National End of Life Care Programme, 2010). Patients with cancer and who are younger (less than 45 years old) account for the majority of the home and hospice deaths, which means that although most people die of something other than cancer and when they are old, the likelihood of a home death for these individuals is very low (Gomes and Higginson, 2008). Gomes and Higginson's (2008) comprehensive analysis of mortality statistics over the past 30 years shows that the proportion of home deaths has steadily decreased from 31.1% in 1974 to 18.1% in 2003. If this trend continues, then by 2030 only one in ten deaths will occur at home, which, coupled with an increasing death rate after 2012 due to the baby boomers reaching very old age, will result in a need for expanding inpatient facilities by more than 20%. However, most agree that hospital, with its focus on interventional medicine, is not the best place to be for high-quality end-of-life care, so this expansion of services for the dying is needed in hospices and care homes. If reducing hospital inpatient deaths could be achieved, then a great deal more support will be needed in the community to help families care for the dying. Gomes and Higginson calculate that if support from community health and social services for care of the dying was doubled, then the proportion of deaths at home could be one in three in 2012 instead of the current value of less than one in five.

There are many complex reasons for the changes over the last few decades in where people die. For example, there is an increasing number of people living alone, which means there is no one else at home to provide care (Grundy *et al*, 2004). General practitioners make fewer home visits than they did 30 years ago and this has resulted in more hospitalisations (Gomes, 2006, cited in Gomes and Higginson, 2008). For older people, too, the availability of informal (family) caregivers may be limited, and their concern for the burden caregiving places on family members may also be a reason for older people dying in hospital (Patrick *et al*, 2001; Vig *et al*, 2002). As a result of changes in society, the conventional ideal of a good death is difficult to achieve. What is important to know is what people want when it comes to care at the end of life. Sutton and Coast (2006) reviewed the literature in relation to older people's preferences at the end of life and found three main areas of focus in the research: treatment decisions; the good death; and place of care/death. The idea of what is a good death is particularly important in getting to the heart of understanding what people think respecting dignity at the end of life really means in practice.

PREFERENCES FOR END-OF-LIFE CARE

The idea of a good death is a widespread concept but it varies culturally and has its roots in social history (Seale, 1998; Walters, 2004). Our current 'western' view of a good death has evolved from influences in the recent past. From a health perspective, there has been a transition from acute conditions to chronic conditions as the predominant problem, a transition that has diminished some of the reality of death by changing illness from being life threatening to life limiting. From a health service perspective, care has been institutionalised away from the home and into acute hospitals as care has become more professionalised and technology based. Furthermore, the advances in technology in healthcare have emphasised the importance of restorative and 'heroic' interventions to the exclusion of other goals of care. These changes have not only resulted in people becoming distanced from the experience of caring for a dying relative or friend, but have also resulted in death being seen as failure and something preventable or at least able to be postponed (Christakis, 1999; Timmermans, 2005).

Similarly the euthanasia debate, including the use of so-called 'physician-assisted suicide', influences people's ideas about options at the end of life. On one side it is suggested that to take control of the timing of death before one's quality of life is too greatly impaired represents a good death, allowing one to die with dignity. On the other side, the management of suffering at the end of life through expert palliative care is offered as a way to maintain dignity and remove the need to end one's life (Materstvedt *et al*, 2003). Needless to say, these are essentially contested concepts and thus neither side will win the argument or convince the other side to alter their views, since they are based on values and not facts (Gallie, 1955–1956). The scare tactics of some activists that old people will be euthanised unwillingly and the current limited access to specialist palliative care make both these arguments a source of concern rather than a solution. Another 'western' trend, connected with the self-determination element of the euthanasia debate and which has influenced the social perception of a good death, has developed out of the rise of individualism in the pursuit of happiness and success. This is reflected in bioethics as we see that autonomy is given more importance over the other main bioethics principles of non-maleficence (do no harm), beneficence (do good) and justice (Beauchamp and Childress, 2008; Tsai, 2008).

Out of these influences, what appears to be important in terms of dignity is how we define personhood. Being a person is being someone who is rational, self-aware, and capable of valuing their own life, entitled to freedom and therefore having the right to make choices for themselves (Locke, 1964; Tsai, 2008). This western view of human personhood and the right to be treated with dignity can be supplemented by an 'eastern' view of personhood. Tsai (2008) explains that there are two layers of personhood in Confucian philosophy. In addition to the autonomous self, personhood also relies on one's relationships and support of others, particularly family and community. This is an interesting addition to understanding personhood, which is not absent from the way ordinary western people think but has certainly not been included explicitly in formal philosophical and ethical definitions.

These social and historical influences are reflected in older people's views on preferences for end-of-life care. Sutton and Coast's (2006) review identified the main preferences of older adults, which are summarised in Box 10.1.

BOX 10.1 *Summary of preferences at the end of life*

➤ To have family and friends present during the dying process and at the end
➤ To be pain free and have symptoms managed effectively
➤ To be treated as a whole person, including psychospiritual support
➤ To be prepared for death
➤ To maintain independence and control over activities and care
➤ To be able to access well-coordinated care services
➤ To be cared for and to die in the place of choice

These points illustrate an integration of the elements of personhood as already presented. Clearly people are connected with their families and friends, and maintaining relationships is very important. Being treated as a whole person, and having symptoms attended to in order to maintain a sense of self and control over one's body is also necessary for personhood. Being prepared for death and maintaining independence are both related to control and can be interpreted as the continuation of adult life where the person had autonomy and conducted their affairs independently. The final two items can be viewed together, since the ability to be cared for and to die in the place of choice is reliant on access to services that meet the needs of the patient and family.

These are the important features that, if present or managed will facilitate the best death possible. They are also the same factors that promote dignity for the individual. Definitions of dignity related to healthcare incorporate a few agreed concepts. Dignity is an innate or intrinsic part of being human and is related to self-esteem and social roles (Sandman, 2002; Badcott, 2003). Furthermore, dignity is manifested through our personal behaviour (Jacelon, 2003) and in the way we recognise the dignity in others (Pleschberger, 2007).

The central idea of the behavioural component is that an action 'shows respect' either to oneself or to others. If dignity is known through human behaviour then it must be learned, and that suggests also that there may be cultural differences in how dignity is expressed. Nordenfelt's (2004) typology of dignity (*see* previous discussions in Chapters 2, 3 and 9) is of use to us here in that two of the four types of dignity he defines are particularly important in the care of the dying: the dignity of *Menschenwürde* (the German term for dignity attributed simply because we are human) and the dignity of personal identity.

As Wainwright and Gallagher (2008) ably argue, nurses have unparalleled opportunity to demonstrate respect for life, not just in saving life but in protecting patients' vulnerability to the embarrassment and humiliation that can so readily accompany healthcare interventions. The dignity of personal identity carries with it considerable risk of loss since it relates to self-respect and concepts like integrity, autonomy and inclusion. When patients are unconscious, cognitively impaired or indeed so close to death that they are unresponsive, then these virtues associated with dignity have disappeared. As nurses, though, the dignity of *Menschenwürde* means that we will treat these people with all due respect despite their having lost elements of personal identity and personhood as formally defined.

Dying is a very problematic concept in relation to dignity because everything that points to the attributes of personhood and therefore to commanding respect for personal dignity is at risk. In all other areas of healthcare, restoration of personhood and dignity is a foreseeable and achievable goal as the aim of treatment and invasive procedures is recovery. During these periods of vulnerability, dignity can be palliated by the actions and communications of health professionals. For example, providing privacy, being respectful in communication and giving patients as much choice as possible help people retain their dignity and personhood despite their vulnerabilities. In healthcare in general, any loss of personhood and dignity can be seen as transitory. But with dying, the real and present threat of non-existence, of non-personhood, makes the risk to dignity greater than at any other time in life. The fear of an undignified dying is magnified by the grief not only of losing autonomy and freedom during the dying process, but of losing self entirely. Thus the need to be treated with respect is even more important at the end of life.

FACILITATING DIGNIFIED DYING

The statistical picture painted above, alongside the areas of preference for a good death, suggests that we are not doing very well at facilitating end-of-life care in the way that patients say they want it. Since the early 2000s, the Department of Health has had an increasing policy focus on end-of-life care in the UK which aims to promote patient choice, support end-of-life care in the community and ensure that not just cancer patients get a 'Rolls Royce' service (Clark *et al*, 2005). But the reality of caring for the dying comes down to the individuals who attend to that person and family. No policy, however well thought through and implemented, can substitute for excellent, compassionate care by well-educated professional nurses who provide a person-centred, evidence-based approach to their work.

This section of the chapter is divided into two parts. First we will explore the nature of suffering, which is the antithesis to dignity, and how dignified dying may provide a better alternative for approaching the care of the dying. Then we will examine the interventions designed to facilitate dignified dying, before concluding the chapter.

Dignity and suffering

Understanding what dignity is at the end of life, from the dying person's perspective, is a fundamental step toward facilitating dignified dying. Several studies have shown that the descriptors of personhood and dignity as described above hold true for the dying person. Self-image, self-determination and a sense of personal identity remain important (Chochinov *et al*, 2002; Ternestedt *et al*, 2002; Enes Duartes, 2003; Pleschberger, 2007). The centrality of social relationships is also confirmed as essential to dignity at the end of life (Street, 2001; Ternestedt *et al*, 2002; Enes Duartes, 2003; Pleschberger, 2007). However, the impact of the body's deterioration is a feature that is particular to dignity in the dying person. Street (2001) suggests that dignity is embodied as it is found to be so related to the loss of bodily function and process of decay associated with dying. Similarly, in the work of Franklin *et al* (2006), the themes revealed that the greatest threats to dignity were the 'unrecognizable body' and 'fragility and dependency', both starkly revealed by the process of dying. The connection between the dying body and loss of dignity clearly directs us to provide comfort through managing the physical as well as psychological, social and spiritual needs, in order to maintain dignity and prevent or minimise suffering.

Suffering and dignity are integrated concepts, particularly at the end of life or in life-threatening situations. Not only does suffering cause loss of dignity but it is also the case that a loss of dignity causes suffering. The fear of dying often relates to the desire not to suffer and this fear of suffering is at the core of the problems associated with the end of life. The fear of suffering itself causes suffering. Suffering is a complex, multidimensional and subjective concept that varies in intensity, severity and bearability (Ruijs *et al*, 2009). Despite its persistent presence with health-related problems, suffering has not been well described from the patient's point of view.

Ruijs *et al* (2009) attempted to conceptualise and measure unbearable suffering by developing a questionnaire based on the elements of suffering identified from research in health professionals' views of suffering. The 69 items fall into five domains: medical signs and symptoms (37 items); loss of function (seven items); personal aspects (17 items); social and environmental aspects (six items); and nature and prognosis of disease (two items). Participants were asked to rate not only the severity of each item but also the degree of unbearable-ness. The fifth domain on the nature and prognosis of disease asks patients to rate two interesting statements, one on the 'fear of future suffering' and the second on the 'fear of not any longer having the strength to bear the suffering' (p.4). The analysis showed strong relationships between presence and bearability, supporting the idea that relieving symptoms or concerns in one domain may result in an increase in the availability of capacity to bear suffering within that domain or perhaps in other domains.

Similarly, Chochinov and colleagues considered the relationship between suffering and dignity, developing from that the dignity model as an empirically testable approach to intervening rather than measuring suffering (Chochinov *et al*, 2002, 2008). The components of the model are: illness-related concerns – including level of independence and symptom distress; dignity-conserving repertoire – including dignity-conserving perspectives and practices; and the social dignity inventory – including privacy boundaries, social support, care tenor (attitude and approach of staff), burden to others, and aftermath concerns (concerns about what will happen after death).

Kolcaba's work on the theory of comfort in nursing also provides some insight (Kolcaba, 2009). She suggests that there are three levels of comfort outcomes: to relieve discomfort, to ease discomfort or to transcend discomfort. These goals work well with the concept of suffering at the end of life in that it may be possible to relieve completely some forms of suffering and to ease to some degree other forms of suffering. However, sometimes it is necessary to assist patients and families in transcending, rising above, the suffering and supporting them to find some level of comfort in very discomforting situations. In Kolcaba's theory, discomfort can be experienced in three domains: physical, psychospiritual and environmental. These are not dissimilar domains to those of Ruijs *et al*'s (2009) work on suffering or Chochinov *et al*'s (2002) work on dignity, and confirm the hypothesis that suffering and comfort, and therefore dignity, are all multidimensional, whole-person experiences. Furthermore, these three theoretical views highlight that the relationship between suffering and dignity can be balanced by comfort. Taking these three related concepts together, one can see how comfort measures counteract the effects of suffering and promote dignity.

Interventions for dignified dying

The term 'dignified dying' has only appeared in the nursing literature in the past five years. It is an important component of a good death, since dignity figures highly in the construction of a good death for most people. The good death poses some problems in that there is a tendency to have a rigid, idealised view of what is a good death, and if those components are not there, then the circumstances of the death can be construed as a failure of care (Walters, 2004). For example, many nurses both in the community and in hospital value a home death over and above all other considerations, so much so that they believe they have failed if the patient is moved to hospital; thus a good death could not be achieved even if the family is relieved and the patient's pain is better managed in hospital (Smith and Porock, 2010). The professionals' view of what constitutes a good death can sometimes be in conflict with what patients and families want or need and families can feel under pressure to comply with what professionals consider to be a good death (Walters, 2004).

The dying scene is idealised in a good death scenario, in a similar way that the birth plan for the delivery of a baby can be idealised. When things do not go quite to plan with the delivery, there can be great disappointment, guilt and grief. With dignified dying, the aim is simply to ensure the patients' and families' dignity throughout the process, whatever that may entail, wherever it may occur. For the dying person and family, the intention may be to die at home but because of unfamiliarity with the dying process, and with the success of medical treatment, this sometimes does not happen. For example, over the last year or so of the patient's life when a crisis has occurred, such as an infection or uncontrolled pain, the patient has gone to hospital, been treated, and gone home again. The family is not to know that this time it is the terminal event. So they go to hospital with the patient fully expecting sufficient recovery to go home, albeit aware that the patient will die at home. When the infection or metabolic crisis cannot be reversed, the patient then enters the active phase of dying but is not in the place of choice. The idealised death scene has to be abandoned and the patient and family begin to face uncharted and unprepared-for waters. Thus, dignified dying provides a way of thinking about facilitating the best death possible for both the patient and family without the constraints of the idealised good death.

As we have seen, dignity is a multidimensional, subjective concept; therefore, multidimensional and dynamic interventions are needed as solutions when dignity is threatened by suffering at the end of life. Physical suffering is probably the area of palliative care specialty that is best developed and most widely recognised. The assessment and management of pain in particular are critical to dignity-preserving care. Psychological, social, spiritual and existential suffering is less well understood and not amenable to intervention or management – at least not in the same way that physical symptoms are. For example, there is no dose, route or frequency of administration for a social intervention. Chochinov (2006) notes that many of the interventions for dignity that have been noted would be categorised as 'niceties' of care or 'touchy-feely', but emphasises the centrality of these actions and interactions as of the highest priority if we are to maintain and support dignity at the end of life. Fundamental to providing dignity-preserving care is finding out who the patient is, what is important to them and what they value. This is the assessment process for dignity. From that, creative and individual care can be designed. The simple act of recognising the suffering as experienced by the patient, validating that experience as real, is in itself a dignity-preserving intervention. As Chochinov (2006) states, '. . . patients are looking for affirmation regarding their sense of worth in spite of their dyspnoea, incontinence and disfigurement' (p.94).

Suffering cannot be palliated in the same way as pain at the end of life. Rather than masking with analgesia or sedation, as is acceptable and effective with physical pain, the issues underlying psychological, social and spiritual and existential suffering should be explored and, as far as possible, resolved. Rousseau (2000) suggests the following dignity-preserving activities in addition to controlling symptoms and providing supportive presence: use life review to recognise purpose, value and meaning in life and in dying; explore guilt, remorse, forgiveness and reconciliation; and facilitate religious expression and focus on meditative practices that promote healing rather than cure. These interventions require great skill and courage, particularly in a healthcare system where these activities are not valued or built into the workload. However, health professionals caring for the dying must not shy away from allowing the patient time to express their concerns, or from supporting family members wherever possible in this process, as well as facilitating access to those who can support more in-depth exploration.

Kissane (2001) uses the term 'demoralising syndrome' to describe the impact of suffering on dignity. His suggestions for care are very similar to Rousseau's and Chochinov's but he adds the importance of balancing support for grief with the promotion of hope and suggests that continuity of care is essential to providing this kind of support. Hopelessness is highly correlated with suicidal ideation and desire for death, more so than depression (Chochinov *et al*, 1998), and fundamentally undermines the sense that life has any value or worth (Chochinov, 2006). It might seem difficult, if not impossible, to find hope at the end of life. However, the key is in reframing what is hoped for. Hope is a way of coping, a way of enduring suffering. Patients may hope for no more suffering, or for living each day, or for a peaceful death and they may hope for their family's future (Duggleby, 2000; Duggleby and Wright, 2004).

Dignity therapy is a specific technique developed and tested by Chochinov and colleagues (2005), which focuses on finding meaning. Patients are asked to relate the elements of their personal history that they most want to be remembered or to focus on things that they feel must be said. The sessions are recorded and then transcribed and presented back to the patient who can then distribute them to family members. The impact of this simple act is profound as it provides comfort to relatives and generates a tangible legacy for the patient. Measuring the impact has shown improvements in depressive symptoms and desire for death.

Fear of the dying process is part of psychological suffering and it can be experienced by family as well as patients. As with the fear of any new experience, education and support are of vital importance. Teaching patients and families about the dying process may seem a daunting prospect but is essential for dignified dying. Many hospices and palliative care services provide descriptions of the final hours and days of life so that fear of the unknown can be reduced. Many services have these descriptions on line and they are well-accessed sites. Teaching about the dying process has been recognised as part of family care and has been confirmed, along with privacy for the family and encouraging involvement in care, in several countries as a positive intervention for dignified dying (Wilson *et al*, 2006; Coenen *et al*, 2007).

Privacy is often connected with dignity but listed as if they were separate concepts. Privacy is a part of dignity and it is important to consider this element in more detail. The home death is appealing in part because of its ability to keep the dying process private. Dying in a public place is not part of the idealised death. In their critical look at end-of-life care at home, Exley and Allen (2007) describe the institutionalisation and medicalisation of the home where the sick room takes on the appearance, and sometimes the routine, of the hospital. Although this is probably not what people have in mind with a home death, it does afford one feature not always present in hospital and that is privacy from other patients and relatives. Porock *et al* (2009) provide an explicit description of the lack of privacy for dying people in general hospitals in the UK. An extract from this work is presented in Box 10.2. The field note extract relates to a situation where an older patient's two daughters arrived on the ward and a nurse asked the doctor to speak to them about their mother's condition. There followed a conversation in the ward with the daughters sitting at a table, a cleaner nearby, and several doctors and a nurse standing by the daughters. The doctor explained to the patient's daughters that most older people with dementia die of pneumonia rather than their dementia. He then asked them how they wished their mother to be treated, pointing out that there were very limited choices. As you read in Box 10.2, not only was there a lack of privacy but the staff apparently displayed a lack of empathy for the patient's daughters.

Providing privacy is more than just pulling a curtain around the bed. The impact of watching another patient dying on those sharing a bay is raised in Porock *et al*'s work, but more research is needed to really understand the implications and be able to act effectively on patients' behalf. Dilemmas between the idealised good death being facilitated by offering a single room and the desire not to hide away the dying was another feature of providing end-of-life care in such a public arena. Street and Love (2005) attend to the issue of privacy

BOX 10.2 *Field note extract from 'Dying in public: the nature of dying in a public hospital'*

Daughters' eyes begin to well up. One states clearly that they do not want any heroics if their mother has a heart attack, and that this has already been decided. She wants to know what the options are. Doctor suggests that it may be kindest to allow the mother to die in peace with no pain rather than continue with active treatment (antibiotics). Daughters both agree but they want her fed to the end and kept pain free. Doctor states that he will note their wishes. This seems a very private conversation to have in the middle of a busy ward with trolleys and cleaners all around. The daughters are left welling up and go to see their mum. No assistance is offered by staff for chairs or cup of tea or anything remotely empathic. Both daughters are clearly fighting back the tears on seeing their mum in bed. The ward round continues in this bay with this family left exposed in the rawness of their newly realised embarkation on a journey toward the loss of their mother. It is surreal and yet ordinary.

(Porock *et al*, 2009, p.16, reprinted by permission of the publisher Taylor & Francis Group, www.informaworld.com)

BOX 10.3 *Characteristics of dignified dying, adapted from Wilson et al (2006), p.38*

➤ Verbalises relief of pain
➤ Expresses control of symptoms
➤ Participates in decisions for care and treatment
➤ Verbalises physical comfort
➤ Verbalises spiritual contentment
➤ Reviews life experiences
➤ Resolves personal and family concerns
➤ Feelings of sorrow, grief and detachment processed through mourning
➤ Expresses feelings of loss
➤ Consciously dealing with emotions relating to impending death
➤ Shares feelings of loss with significant others
➤ Expresses spiritual concerns
➤ Expresses expectations about the impending end of life
➤ Expresses acceptance of dying
➤ Verbalises any lack of control in treatment decisions
➤ Verbalises any lack of respect from healthcare providers

and caution us to consider privacy not just in terms of environment but also in terms of psychosocial and moral dimensions. Providing privacy as a means of preserving dignity is an essential intervention in care of the dying.

With all interventions, it is important to evaluate and determine their effectiveness. The concept of dignified dying is being developed and tested as a nursing diagnosis. Wilson *et al* (2006) suggest 16 characteristics that would indicate that the patient's dignity is maintained. These are listed in Box 10.3.

These are helpful indicators of dignified dying but they do rely on the patient being sufficiently cognitively intact and assertive, particularly with professional caregivers, and that might not be the case. It also assumes that acceptance is a necessary part of dignified dying when clearly there are many examples of patients who at best may be feeling resigned to the fact of their impending death but not really prepared to accept it (Walters, 2004). These feelings are also legitimate and need to be accepted as part of the human experience at the end of life. Dignified dying cannot be any more uniform than the idealised 'good death', as that would inhibit the individual's own expression of dignity.

What is similar about all dignity-preserving interventions is the need not only for presence and time but also for the courage to spend time with a person who is dying, an activity that can seriously challenge our own sense of stability and ability to cope with our own mortality. Thus an important intervention for dignity-preserving care is for professional and family caregivers to be cared for and supported themselves.

CONCLUSION

This chapter has reviewed death in our society in terms of where and when people die, and has explored the preferences for end-of-life care, particularly in older adults, in order to provide a context for understanding dignity at the end of life and how to facilitate dignified dying. Facilitating dignified dying through dignity-preserving strategies is an achievable goal. It takes the courage to talk to people about their deaths and is contingent on the recognition and open awareness of death. Providing end-of-life care that preserves dignity is not an easy area of care but it is a privilege and one that can be immensely rewarding and life affirming. NB: Chapter 11 (Community care and dignity) includes exploration of a community-based case study of end-of-life care.

REFERENCES

Badcott D (2003) The basis and relevance of emotional dignity. *Medicine Health Care and Philosophy* 6: 123–31.

Beauchamp TL, Childress JF (2008) *Principles of Biomedical Ethics* (6e). London: Oxford University Press.

Chochinov HM (2006) Dying, dignity and new horizons in palliative end-of-life care. *CA: A Cancer Journal for Clinicians* 5: 84–103.

Chochinov HM, Wilson KG, Enns M *et al* (1998) Depression, hopelessness and suicidal ideation in the terminally ill. *Psychosomatics* 39: 366–70.

Chochinov HM, Hack T, Hassard T *et al* (2002) Dignity in the terminally ill: a cross-sectional cohort study. *Lancet* 360: 2026–30.

Chochinov HM, Hack T, Hassard T *et al* (2005) Dignity therapy: a novel psychotherapeutic intervention for patients nearing death. *Journal of Clinical Oncology* 23: 5520–5.

Chochinov HM, Hassard T, McClement S *et al* (2008) The patient dignity inventory: a novel way of measuring dignity-related distress in palliative care. *Journal of Pain and Symptom Management* 36(6): 559–71.

Christakis N (1999) *Death Foretold: prophecy and prognosis in medical care.* Chicago, IL: University of Chicago Press.

Clark D, Small N, Wright M *et al* (2005) *A Bit of Heaven for the Few? An oral history of the modern hospice movement in the United Kingdom.* Lancaster: Observatory Publications.

Coenen A, Doorenbos A, Wilson SA (2007) Nursing interventions to promote dignified dying in four countries. *Oncology Nursing Forum* 34(6): 1151–6.

Department of Health (2005) *The National Service Framework for Long-term Conditions.* London: HMSO.

Douglas K (2004) Death defying. *New Scientist* 28 **August**: 40–3.

Duggleby W (2000) Enduring suffering: a grounded theory analysis of the pain experience of elderly hospice patients with cancer. *Oncology Nursing Forum* 27: 825–30.

Duggleby W, Wright K (2004) Elderly palliative care patients' descriptions of hope-fostering strategies. *International Journal of Palliative Nursing* 10: 352–9.

Enes Duartes SP (2003) An exploration of dignity in palliative care. *Palliative Medicine* 17: 263–9.

Exley C, Allen D (2007) A critical examination of home care: end of life care as an illustrative case. *Social Science and Medicine* 65(11): 2317–27.

Franklin L-L, Ternestedt B-M, Nordenfelt L (2006) Views on dignity of elderly nursing home residents. *Nursing Ethics* 13(2): 130–46.

Gallie WB (1955–1956) Essentially contested concepts. *Proceedings of the Aristotelian Society, New Series* 56: 167–98.

Gomes B, Higginson IJ (2008) Where people die (1974–2030): past trends, future projections and implications for care. *Palliative Medicine* 22: 33–41.

Grundy E, Mayer D, Young H *et al* (2004) Living arrangements and place of death of older people with cancer in England and Wales: a record linkage study. *British Journal of Cancer* 91(5): 907–12.

Higginson IJ, Astin P, Dolan S (1998) Where do cancer patients die? Ten year trends in the place of death of cancer patients in England. *Palliative Medicine* 12: 353–63.

Hopkinson J, Hallet C, Luker K (2003) Caring for dying people in hospital. *Journal of Advanced Nursing* 44(5): 525–33.

Jacelon CS (2003) The dignity of elders in an acute care setting. *Qualitative Health Research* 13(4): 543–56.

Kissane DW (2001) Demoralization: its impact on informed consent and medical care. *Medical Journal of Australia* 175: 537–39.

Kolcaba C (2009) Comfort. In: Peterson SJ, Bredow TS (eds) *Middle Range Theories.*

Application to nursing research (2e). Philadelphia: Lippincott Williams and Wilkins, pp.254–70.

Locke J (1964) *An Essay Concerning Human Understanding Book 2.* London: Oxford University Press.

Materstvedt LJ, Clark D, Ellershaw J *et al* (2003) Euthanasia and physician-assisted suicide: a view from an EAPC Ethics Task Force. *Palliative Medicine* **17**: 97–101.

National End of Life Care Programme (2010) *Variations in Place of Death in England. Inequalities or appropriate consequences of age, gender and cause of death?* London: NHS.

Nordenfelt L (2004) The varieties of dignity. *Health Care Analysis* **12**(20): 69–89.

Office for National Statistics (2009) www.statistics.gov.uk/downloads/theme_health/dr2009/dr-09.pdf (accessed 26 October 2010).

Patrick DL, Engelberg RA, Curtis JR (2001) Evaluating the quality of dying and death. *Journal of Pain and Symptom Management* **22**(3): 717–26.

Pfund R, Fowler-Kerry S (2010) *Perspectives on Palliative Care for Children and Young People: a global discourse.* Oxford: Radcliffe Publishing.

Pleschberger S (2007) Dignity and the challenge of dying in nursing homes: the residents' view. *Age and Ageing* **36**: 197–202.

Porock D, Pollock K, Jurgens F (2009) Dying in public: the nature of dying in an acute hospital setting. *Journal of Housing for the Elderly* **23**(1): 10–28.

Rousseau P (2000) Spirituality and the dying patient. *Journal of Clinical Oncology* **18**: 2000–2002.

Ruijs KDM, Onwuteaka-Philipsen BD, van der Wal G *et al* (2009) Unbearability of suffering at the end of life: the development of a new measuring device, the SOS-V. *Biomed Central Palliative Care* **8**(16). www.biomedcentral.com/1472-684X/8/16 (accessed 12 October 2010).

Sandman L (2002) What's the use of human dignity within palliative care? *Nursing Philosophy* **3**: 177–81.

Seale C (1998) *Constructing Death: the Sociology of Dying and Bereavement.* Cambridge: Cambridge University Press.

Shipman C, Higginson IJ, White P *et al* (2007) *Scoping Exercise on Generalist Services for Adults at the End of Life: research, knowledge, policy and future research needs. Report 3: the consultation report for the National Co-ordinating Centre for NHS Service Delivery and Organisation R&D (NCCSDO).* London: King's College London.

Smith R, Porock D (2010) Caring for people dying at home: a research study into the needs of community nurses. *International Journal of Palliative Nursing* **15**(12): 601–8.

Street A (2001) Constructions of dignity in end-of-life care. *Journal of Palliative Care* **17**(2): 93–101.

Street AF, Love A (2005) Dimensions of privacy in palliative care: views of health professionals. *Social Science and Medicine* **60**: 1795–1804.

Sutton E, Coast J (2006) Older people's preferences at the end of life: a review of the literature. In: Woodthorpe K (ed) *Layers of Dying and Death: papers presented at the 4th Global Conference of Dying and Death. Wed 12th–Friday 14th July 2006. Mansfield College, Oxford.* Oxford: Inter-Disciplinary Press.

Ternestedt B-M, Andershed B, Eriksson M *et al* (2002) A good death: development of a nursing model of care. *Journal of Hospice and Palliative Nursing* **3**: 153–60.

Timmermans S (2005) Death brokering: constructing culturally appropriate deaths. *Sociology of Health and Illness* **27**: 993–1013.

Tsai DF-C (2008) Personhood and autonomy in multicultural health care settings. *American Medical Association Journal of Ethics* **10**(3): 171–6.

Vig EK, Davenort NA, Pearlman RA (2002) Good deaths, bad deaths and preferences for the end of life: a qualitative study of geriatric outpatients. *Journal of the American Geriatrics Society* **50**(9): 1541–8.

Wainwright P, Gallagher A (2008) On different types of dignity in nursing care: a critique of Nordenfelt. *Nursing Philosophy* **9**: 46–54.

Walters G (2004) Is there such a thing as a good death? *Palliative Medicine* **18**(5): 404–408.

Wilson SA, Coenen A, Doorenbos A (2006) Dignified dying as a phenomenon in the United States. *Journal of Hospice and Palliative Nursing* **8**(1): 34–41.

CHAPTER 11

Community care and dignity

Candice Pellett

INTRODUCTION

People live their lives primarily in their own homes and communities, where their health and well-being are influenced by the events in which they find themselves involved. Primary care is diverse and can be complicated, with a vast and increasing range of care, treatments and support being delivered in the community setting. This chapter will explore issues relating to dignity in care for patients in the community in the United Kingdom (UK). Care delivery by the district nursing team in patients' own homes, residential homes and clinics will be focused on, though the principles discussed apply to other healthcare professionals working in the community, and indeed will be relevant in other countries too.

Community staff often work with patients and their families over a long period of time, so it is imperative to build trusting relationships to promote, where possible, independence, choice and empowerment along their healthcare journey. Lack of respect for people's dignity can take many forms and may be experienced differently from person to person. Dignity should permeate care delivery and includes people having choices about how their care is delivered and having their religious and cultural needs considered.

This chapter includes case studies that focus on the dignity of patients at the end of their lives, patients requiring wound care, and adults with long-term conditions, as these are all situations commonly encountered in community care. The case studies are based on the author's practice experience; all patients' names and identifying features have been altered to maintain anonymity.

LEARNING OUTCOMES

By the end of the chapter you will be able to:
➤ discuss the context of dignity in community care, with reference to current UK health policy and the district nursing team
➤ identify key principles relating to dignity within patients' own homes and residential settings

➤ explain how the district nursing team can promote dignity for patients in the community, with specific reference to patients with chronic wounds, patients undergoing palliative care and patients with long-term conditions.

DIGNITY IN COMMUNITY CARE: THE CONTEXT

Dignity is important to every individual, irrespective of the situation and the healthcare setting in which they find themselves. Increasingly, care takes place in the community rather than in hospital; indeed, in the UK, 90% of people accessing healthcare do so in primary and community settings (Darzi, 2009). *Our Health, Our Care, Our Say* (Department of Health [DH], 2006) asserted that healthcare is shifting from hospital to primary care across the health spectrum, from complex disease management to end-of-life care, giving patients and carers preference where possible to be treated closer to home. The DH (2006) discussed the importance of supporting and caring for people at home, particularly those aged over 65 years and those with long-term conditions. This was further supported by *High Quality Care for All* (DH, 2008a), which sets out the vision for a modern, responsive, high-quality service delivered to people nearer to home and aimed at preventing unnecessary hospital admissions. Furthermore, services should focus on the importance of patients' experiences in terms of quality of care and caring, which includes 'compassion, dignity and respect with which patients are treated' (DH, 2008a, p.47). These principles should be applied across all settings within the community, including general practitioners' (GPs') surgeries, health clinics, community hospitals and within patients' own homes.

In the UK, community care is usually led by district nurses (DNs) for people who require nursing in their own homes. DNs hold a post-registration specialist practitioner qualification and are responsible for the delivery of patient and carer-centred care. DN team members may include registered nurses and healthcare support workers who have a wide range of skills. DNs are usually attached to GPs and cover a defined geographical area. They provide care to patients aged 16 years and over who are registered with the practice and who are usually confined to their home or live in a residential setting. The DN service provides care 365 days per year, and in many parts of the UK there is 24 hour support. Visits are often on a regular basis and over a long period of time; therefore, DNs are in a position to accurately assess the needs of the patient and their family. With health policy aiming to provide care closer to home, the DN service is rapidly taking on ever-increasing roles as more complex care is delivered in the community, whether managing long-term conditions, preventing unnecessary emergency admissions or delivering end-of-life care. The team is well placed to liaise across the boundaries of primary and acute services, working with all professionals involved in patients' care pathways to maximise and coordinate care to deliver a high-quality service. Maintaining patient dignity is central to good community nursing practice, particularly as DNs often care for patients at a vulnerable time in their lives.

The fundamental role and responsibility of the DN service are to offer full holistic assessment of patients in addition to recognising their carers' needs, and to provide skilled nursing care to meet assessed needs. The service endeavours to empower patients and their carers by working in partnership and where possible, promoting independence. The skills offered by the DN team include assessment, planning, implementing and evaluating the needs of the patients and their carers/families within their own homes. This may include assessment and treatment of incontinence and assessment and prescribing of equipment to facilitate care in patients' homes, thus enabling individuals to maximise their quality of life within the limits of their illness or disease, or to enable a full recovery. DNs use personalised care planning with patients, rather than setting patients' goals for them, thus actively involving patients in deciding, agreeing and owning how their health will be managed, promoting choice and enhancing dignity. This philosophy is supported by the Government's principle of shared decision making of 'no decision about me without me' (p.13) which involves patients working in partnership with clinicians in choosing their care and treatments that will improve their health outcomes (DH, 2010).

DIGNITY IN PEOPLE'S OWN HOMES

District nursing teams undertake the majority of care in patients' own homes; therefore, they are 'guests' in the patients' environment. Nurses and other healthcare professionals are there by the patient's invitation and consent and often have information and knowledge about the patient, their family and their lifestyle. Therefore, confidentiality of information is paramount, including that relating to the patient's health, values, beliefs, home environment, finances and relationships. This information must be treated with respect for the patient's and their family's right to privacy, as otherwise dignity will be compromised. Some communities, especially in village settings, are very close-knit and it can sometimes be difficult to maintain confidentiality when the nurse works and lives in the same environment. Relatives, friends or neighbours of the patient may ask for information without the patient's knowledge or consent and may become quite affronted when the community team is unable to answer their questions. However, information about patients is private and nurses have a duty of confidentiality to respect and protect their patient (Nursing and Midwifery Council [NMC], 2008), as do other healthcare professionals.

The majority of patients on a DN caseload are older people who may be frail and vulnerable, and it is important that they are treated as individuals, valuing them as people who, although they may require support, still have much to give to their families and the wider community. The dignity of older people can easily become compromised as they find themselves in vulnerable situations, often with less control (*see* Chapter 9 for a detailed exploration of dignity and older people). The Royal College of Nursing (2008) suggests that when dignity is present, people feel in control, valued, confident and comfortable and able to make decisions for themselves; however, when dignity is absent, people feel devalued, lacking control and comfort. Being unable to manage and control activities of daily living may have a devastating impact on a person's self-respect and dignity.

When a person requires nursing in their home on a regular basis, they and their family may feel that they lack privacy in many areas of their lives. Dignified care starts when the DN knocks on the door and greets the patient. Asking a person how they would like to be addressed is essential, as a person's name is very personal to them and in some cultures to use a first name as a form of address is considered very disrespectful. Dignity is about respecting the person, which is more than ensuring their physical dignity. It is about maintaining a sense of self-worth, being listened to and being able to make choices about their lives.

Some people require 24-hour care in either their own home or a residential home, and everything they do is open to observation by another person. Conversations, telephone calls, expressions and feelings are on show to others. Personal and intimate care should be sensitively provided to ensure that the dignity of the person remains intact throughout. Attention to preserving privacy and modesty while giving personal care is paramount, as a person's dignity could easily be encroached upon by carelessly exposing their body during intimate care such as undertaking hygiene needs or delivering bowel care. When a person requires help with washing and bathing at home, it is important to ensure that the room door is closed and the window curtains are drawn if the room is overlooked. Staff should also ensure that only the area being washed is uncovered and that the person is warm at all times, which is sometimes difficult to achieve if the bedroom is cold. Often members of the family are present in the house and the person's privacy and dignity should be protected at all times. Consent must be gained from the patient before any discussion about their care takes place when others are present.

DIGNITY IN RESIDENTIAL CARE HOMES

Often people do not want to leave the comfort and privacy of their own homes to live in shared accommodation with strangers. When nursing people living in residential care, it is important to minimise intrusion on their privacy, as they are often in a shared room and they may only be separated from their neighbour by a curtain around the bed. It must be recognised that their room in the residential setting is now their home, so even the most basic step of knocking on the door before entering is important. Bedside curtains may give the illusion of privacy but they do not provide protection from the activities that are occurring behind them. Using a clip or peg to secure the curtain will prevent gaps and remind staff not to enter without warning. The curtains are not smell-proof or sound-proof and it can be very embarrassing when the person is having an enema administered, using the commode or having a bed bath. Respecting a person's privacy and personal space is imperative. Many people are embarrassed if they are moved using a hoist, especially if they wish to use the toilet or commode, and it is important that their clothes are adjusted to ensure that they are not exposed to other residents. An engaged sign on the door will ensure that visitors do not go in and cause embarrassment to the person who is washing or having their wound dressings changed.

To preserve a person's self-respect, it is important to keep their individuality. We must never assume what the patient wants but must respect their individuality at all times. On one occasion, I visited an older person in a residential home to undertake wound dressings and found her crying and withdrawn. After sitting with her, it transpired that it had been her birthday the day before and during tea a carer had placed a large 'top hat' on her head complete with material candles. She would never have agreed to this if she had been asked and felt like she had been treated as a child. The person has since died but her daughter still remembers with sadness how upset her mother had been because she had not been treated as an individual and had felt patronised. It is so important that everyone caring for older people sees beyond a group of residents living in a home and respects them as individuals. All residents are people with life experiences and staff can connect with who they were in the past by using appropriate language and involving them in decision making wherever possible. Dignity must be enforced, not eroded, and at the heart of everything we do, and carers should be seen as expert partners in care rather than controllers of care.

The next sections explore case studies of community patients undergoing wound care, end-of-life care, and care when living with long-term conditions. These case studies illustrate the practical steps that can be taken to promote dignity in community care.

DIGNITY DURING WOUND CARE

Dignity for people undertaking treatments is a basic human right but it is something that could be overlooked in busy clinics. Many leg ulcer clinics are run by DNs in GP surgeries or health clinics. Thousands of people in the UK are affected by leg ulceration, primarily as a consequence of chronic venous insufficiency, with estimated annual costs of care of £200 million (Posnett and Franks, 2007). Essential to patient dignity is promotion of quality of life for individuals, particularly if they have a chronic wound like a leg ulcer, which can often have far-ranging effects on all activities of living. Restrictions in carrying out paid employment, the inability to cope with household activities and loss of mobility can result in loss of control and anxiety and will impact negatively on the patients' quality of life. Various studies have reported the negative impact of leg ulcers on a patient's life (Charles, 1995; Walshe, 1995; Douglas, 2001; Persoon *et al*, 2004).

Reflective activity 11.1 presents questions to help you to consider how a chronic wound affects dignity.

Reflective activity 11.1 The impact of a chronic wound on dignity

If you had a chronic open wound on your lower leg, what impact would this have on your dignity? For example, consider the impact on dignity of:

➤ probable malodour and a constantly oozing wound
➤ associated chronic pain
➤ restricted mobility
➤ having leg bandages in place 24 hours a day.

As you might have considered, malodour from wounds can cause embarrassment for patients and can affect all areas of their lives, causing social isolation and loss of self-esteem. This can be exacerbated when toe-to-knee compression bandaging has to remain in place for up to a week, which may prevent patients from having a shower or bath. Leakage from the ulcer may prevent the person leaving their home between clinic appointments, and cause them to suffer loss of dignity in their outward appearance. A majority of patients experience problems with body image when coping with bandaging. One of the most significant problems that occurs is the visible physical change in the shape and size of the leg, and for some people this necessitates a complete change of preferred style of dress – trousers with wide legs or long skirts are examples of clothing that people with lower leg ulceration adopt whatever their former personal preference. People with oedema to the leg find activities requiring the limb to bend particularly difficult, and swollen and bandaged feet can make shopping for shoes time consuming, costly and depressing. This can have a profound effect on a person's occupation and lifestyle, with feelings of loss of dignity, isolation, anxiety and depression.

The case study in Box 11.1 illustrates the impact of a chronic wound on a patient's dignity and how a DN addressed this situation. As you will read, a crucial factor was listening to Jean's concerns and involving her in planning a solution. Webster and Bryan (2009) found that people value being included in decisions about their care, which allows them to maintain independence and feel more in control about their situation. Although their research was based in a hospital setting, the findings are applicable to the community environment, with the belief that communication is the intervening factor in maintaining control, independence and dignity.

BOX 11.1 *Case study: wound care*

Jean attended an afternoon leg ulcer clinic run by DNs after an absence of some time. She had been referred to the clinic by the practice nurse six months previously, with a venous leg ulcer due to an accidental injury to the lower leg. Walking was a problem due to the increased oedema exacerbated by the failure to wear compression bandaging. Although Jean had been advised on many occasions to maintain good skin care, her skin condition was dry, particularly on her toes and feet. From the documentation it was clear that, gradually, failure to attend the clinics became more frequent despite the DN phoning her and inviting her to attend.

When Jean arrived at the clinic it soon became apparent that she was extremely apprehensive and close to tears, and conversation was difficult. While the nurse was washing Jean's leg she confided that her mother had suffered from leg ulceration due to diabetes which had eventually resulted in amputation of one of her legs. Jean had vivid memories of the discomfort and pain that her mother had experienced and the total loss of dignity and despair she had felt. Jean's situation had brought back all the negative memories of her mother's condition, which had culminated in her not attending the clinics or wearing her bandages. Jean's life was very demanding; combining family commitments and a working day meant she was finding it very difficult to take time off to attend the clinics and she worried that she may lose her job.

After discussions with Jean, the DN suggested that she could attend the evening clinic to have her ulcer redressed by the practice nurse. This enabled Jean to carry on as normal with her employment and maintain control over her day rather than feeling that she was being controlled by her ulcer. Jean's wound healed within ten weeks of attending regular clinic appointments.

DIGNITY IN END-OF-LIFE-CARE

Most deaths occur following long-term illness; according to the DH:

> Around half a million people die in England each year, of which two thirds are aged over 75. The large majority of deaths at the start of the 21st century follow a period of chronic illness such as heart disease, cancer, stroke, chronic respiratory disease, neurological disease or dementia (DH, 2009a, p.123).

Recently, the End of Life Strategy (DH, 2008b), which promotes high-quality care for all adults at the end of life, has stated that most people will spend the majority of the last year of their lives in the community. Therefore, although death itself occurs in hospital for many people (*see* Chapter 10), caring for patients who are dying is a large part of the DN community caseload.

A loss of dignity at the end of life is feared by many people (*see* Chapter 10) and some people feel that lack of support to be able to die in their own home undermines their dignity (Help the Aged, 2007). People must receive excellent care at the end of their lives to give them and their loved ones confidence that they can stay at home if that is their choice. Macleod (2003) suggests that loss of dignity may cause hopelessness, depression and a longing for a quick death. Many people feel that a 'good death' means they have adequate pain relief, privacy, dignity and some control over how and where they die. They may initially receive the bad news of diagnosis in the acute setting, but many aspects of this news and subsequent care are delivered by the primary healthcare team. *Transforming Community Services* (DH, 2009b) suggests the use of an established systematic framework to optimise care delivery. There are best-practice models that aim for dignity as they identify and address people's preferences and needs at the end of life, for example:

➤ *The End of Life Care Transformational Guide* (DH, 2009b)
➤ The Gold Standards Framework (www.goldstandardsframework.nhs.uk)
➤ Liverpool Care Pathway (www.liv.ac.uk/mcpcil/liverpool-care-pathway/)
➤ *Preferred Priorities for Care* (www.endoflifecareforadults.nhs.uk/assets/downloads/ppc.pdf).

The DN service is committed to facilitating patient choice during end-of-life care provision, to allow all patients to die at their preferred place of care with privacy and dignity and with their symptoms controlled. Care includes daily monitoring of a patient's condition, administration of prescribed drugs and assessment of additional support, for example, referral to the Marie Curie service (a UK-based charity delivering home care for people with cancer), and using evidence-based practice in line with national and local policies, guidelines, pathways and protocols. Bereavement visits are also offered to families.

Being involved at the end of someone's life is a privilege. There is only one opportunity to get it right and ensure that the person has a dignified death and their family are well supported. Box 11.2 details a case study as an example of care given to a patient on the DN caseload. As you read the case study of Alan, consider what the community team did to preserve his dignity. A discussion on Alan's care then follows.

BOX 11.2 *Case study: end-of-life care*

Alan was a 73-year-old retired builder who was diagnosed with colorectal carcinoma with lung metastases. He was known to the DNs as they had undertaken flushing of his Hickman line 2 years previously when he was undergoing chemotherapy. As his disease progressed he had been attending a city hospital once weekly for abdominal paracentesis but was finding the sheer effort of travelling to, and waiting for, his treatment more exhausting as his health deteriorated. Alan was placed on the Gold Standard Framework supportive care register. His care plan and needs were discussed at the monthly primary healthcare meetings. Alan's GP and DN were approached by the hospital to discuss the possibility of undertaking ascites drainage at home. Following insertion of a permanent drainage system under local anaesthetic, Alan returned home under the care of the primary healthcare team. Close communication between the DNs, GPs and Macmillan nurse* allowed flexible and timely care to be delivered to Alan when it was appropriate for him.

For the last three months of Alan's life, the nurses visited at least three times a week to assess for re-accumulation of ascites and to observe for abdominal distension and pain. Alan was averaging between 4 and 5 litres drainage per week and was well aware when the drainage needed to be undertaken as he would experience a 'dull, continuous' ache across his abdomen; otherwise he had very little discomfort. He would phone the DN team if extra visits were required to drain the ascitic fluid, thus giving him control of the situation. Alan gradually became more jaundiced and was diagnosed with pruritus. Over time Alan became hypotensive and had increased peripheral oedema. He was eventually placed on the Liverpool Care Pathway and all non-essential medication was stopped. Alan's symptoms were well controlled on a regular prescription administered via a syringe driver. Nursing support was increased to several visits a day. Alan died peacefully within the comfort of his own home in the presence of his family.

*Macmillan nurses are funded by Macmillan Cancer Support, a UK cancer charity.

Discussion

Alan had lived an active, independent life and had found that his advancing illness meant loss of independence and increasing dependence on his wife and health professionals. He initially found this situation very hard to cope with as he felt his freedom of choice and autonomy had diminished. Decision making is the key to our autonomy and determines our lifestyle. Freedom of choice and autonomy are essential components to experiencing dignity. Alan wanted to maintain as much control and choice over his illness and pending death as was possible. Making decisions about our lives, like what to eat and drink, what we wear and whom we choose to live with, is, for most people, something we take for granted and see as a fundamental human right. Nuland (1993) stated that 'The greatest dignity to be found in death is the dignity in the life that preceded it'; therefore, dignity is fundamental in the maintenance of well-being in people who are approaching the end of life.

Over many months, Alan had formed a relationship with the community nursing team as they had been visiting to flush his Hickman line between chemotherapy. A personalised care plan was written that was centred on Alan's needs and concerns and this was shared, with Alan's consent, with every professional involved in his care. As Alan's health eventually deteriorated, his religious and spiritual needs were included in his plan of care. Promoting autonomy of Alan's wishes and values was central to his care delivery and treatment, and respecting his religious needs was essential to maintain his dignity. It is equally important that families and carers feel emotionally supported during end-of-life care delivery. They need confidence to believe that symptoms can be controlled and the dignity of the patient maintained with support from the professionals to help them cope with an acute time of difficulty in their lives.

DIGNITY AND LONG-TERM CONDITIONS

Long-term conditions are described as conditions that currently cannot be cured but can be controlled by medication and other therapies (DH, 2008c). There are approximately 17.5 million people in the UK with a recorded long-term condition and numbers are rising (DH, 2009c). People with a long-term condition want to remain healthy and live independently for as long as possible. Putting people at the heart of their care allows them to make choices about their lives, what is important to them and how they like their care delivered. This can be applied by using a personalised care planning approach to fit in with people's needs, and improvement to the provision of information about long-term conditions to help people manage their own conditions (DH, 2009a). The NHS *Next Stage Review* (DH, 2008d) also suggests that care planning will help to ensure that people with more complex and long-term care needs receive the best, most appropriately tailored package of care to meet their individual needs and requirements. Multidisciplinary team working of nurses, intermediate care and rehabilitation services can support people with long-term conditions to achieve the optimum level of independence for their long-term future.

Box 11.3 provides an example of a man (Tom) living with a long-term condition. As you read the case study, consider the impact of a long-term condition on Tom's dignity, how concurrent social and psychological factors further affect his dignity, and the role of the community team in promoting his dignity. A discussion of Tom's care then follows.

BOX 11.3 *Case study: living with a long-term condition*

Tom lived with his mother who died when he was 56 years of age. He was diagnosed with type 2 diabetes 20 years previously and, due to this condition, was registered blind. Tom has a mild learning disability which means he needs supervision with all his activities of living, including the drawing up and administration of his daily insulin. With DN visits and regular daily visits by carers, Tom managed to remain at home for the next two years. Tom then developed ulcers on both feet, and despite being admitted into a nursing home for care, his skin deteriorated rapidly and a few months later resulted in him having both legs amputated below the knee.

Tom was eventually transferred back to the nursing home but he felt lonely and isolated and he was anxious to return to his own home environment. After several months of rehabilitation, Tom was offered a ground floor apartment in a warden-controlled complex, which he accepted. Tom is totally dependent on others to help him and continues to have daily visits from the DNs to give him his insulin and assess his general health. Agency carers visit every morning to apply Tom's artificial legs, support him with his hygiene needs and prepare his breakfast. Transport collects him every morning to take him to a day centre where he is cared for in a social environment and provided with a hot meal. Carers then visit Tom at his apartment at tea time to prepare his supper, and then again in the early evening to help him prepare for bed. The DNs work closely with the diabetes specialist nurse and GP to monitor Tom's diabetes.

Discussion

As you read, chronic illness and failing health have had an immense impact on Tom's life. He did not want to move out of his home into the nursing home and into unfamiliar surroundings. Being blind made him disorientated and anxious in his new environment. Since Tom has moved into his new flat, he is highly dependent on others for all his needs, and his dignity can very easily be seriously compromised. The timing of visits between carers is crucial for Tom's care planning. If the care agency staff arrive late in the morning Tom gets very upset as he feels 'trapped in his bed' and worries that he won't be ready to go on the transport to the day centre. He says that he cannot make decisions on a day-to-day basis as he is totally dependent on rotas and visits of carers. Tom's feelings of anxiety, helplessness and uncertainty often accompany the reality of total reliance on others. People generally want as much control as possible over their lives. When one is so dependent on others for care, control is easily lost and social isolation and depression are a reality for many people with long-term health conditions. Asking Tom what clothes he would like to wear and what he would like to eat promotes ownership and control that otherwise could easily be compromised. Maintaining privacy and respect are essential aspects of delivering personal care, and matters of personal appearance and hygiene are paramount in preserving dignity.

Tom is confined to bed until the carer attaches his artificial legs, when he can then transfer safely to use the commode. Dignity can be difficult for people who need to use a commode or bedpan (British Geriatrics Society, 2006), and loss of autonomy may result in loss of respect and dignity. In order to maintain dignity, it is suggested by Sturdy (2007, p.9) that healthcare professionals need to 'protect those who are exposed to the alien and often frightening environment of care services'. The DNs who visit Tom are aware that he often needs reassurance and encouragement to boost his confidence with his package of care. Good support is about understanding the needs of the patient, and this can be achieved by working in partnership with them and really listening to their concerns rather than making assumptions about what they want. Communicating effectively with Tom meant that the DN was able to assess his needs and listen to his worries. Finding out details on Tom's daily lifestyle, including what Tom can do for himself and what he cannot manage, built up an overall picture of Tom's life.

Living independently relies on the ability of individuals to carry out a range of personal activities, which can be difficult if there are specific medical conditions. Degeling *et al* (2006) argued that care models must acknowledge the rights and responsibilities of people with long-term conditions to be informed, consulted and included in decision making with their providers of care to determine what they can expect from others and what others can expect from them. Achieving a successful care plan depends on effective communication between all agencies; therefore, the DN liaises regularly with the care agency manager to ensure that Tom's visits are timely. This means that his dignity is not compromised by late visits and stops Tom worrying that he will not be ready for transport every morning, which gives him confidence and reassurance about the coordination of his care plan.

CONCLUSION

As discussed in Chapter 2, dignity can be difficult to define but people know when they have not been treated with respect and dignity. Nurses have a key role in robust care planning for patients in the community environment, whether in a GP surgery, clinic, residential home or the person's own home. Personalising services and listening to what patients really want put them on an equal footing with the professional and allow them control over their lives. All people have histories and lives behind them and hopefully a future too. Shorter futures for older people or people who are near the end of their lives make the time more significant. Working in partnership improves the quality of the patient pathway through joint and effective care planning. Close working with the multidisciplinary team to deliver the care plan helps people maintain optimum functioning, health, well-being, dignity and quality of life. The DH (2009c, p.4) identified that personalised care planning recognises:

> an individual's full range of needs, taking into account their health, personal, family, social, economic, educational, mental health, ethnic and cultural background and circumstances.

People from varying backgrounds may find themselves requiring care in the community setting; therefore, it is imperative that their specific needs are acknowledged. These include the person's ethnic and cultural needs as well as spiritual needs, which are particularly important when delivering end-of-life care. Putting people at the heart of their care allows them to make choices about their lives and express what is important to them. The maintenance of patients' dignity within the community setting is essential to enable the person to feel empowered at a vulnerable time and retain a feeling of control about their care. We all have a duty to deliver dignified care. If dignity is absent then it is very hard to imagine how what is delivered can ever be considered as 'care'.

REFERENCES

British Geriatrics Society (2006) *Dignity Behind Closed Doors.* www.bgs.org.uk/campaigns/dignity.htm (accessed 12 October 2010).

Charles H (1995) The impact of leg ulcers on patients' quality of life. *Professional Nurse* **10**: 571–3.

Darzi A (2009) *Foreword: Transforming Community Services Clinical Guides: ambition, action, achievement.* London: Department of Health, pp.4–5. www.dh.gov.uk/prod_consum_dh/groups/dh_digitalassets/documents/digitalasset/dh_102200.pdf (accessed 12 October 2010).

Degeling P, Close H, Degeling D (2006) *Re-thinking Long Term Conditions. A report on the development and implementation of co-produced, year-based integrated care pathways to improve service provision to people with long term conditions.* Durham: The Centre for Clinical Management Development, Durham University.

Department of Health (2006) *Our Health, Our Care, Our Say: a new direction for community services.* London: Department of Health.

Department of Health (2008a) *High Quality Care for All: NHS next stage review final report*. London: Department of Health.

Department of Health (2008b) *End of Life Strategy: promoting high quality care for all adults at the end of life*. London: Department of Health.

Department of Health (2008c) *Raising the Profile of Long Term Conditions: a compendium of information*. London: Department of Health.

Department of Health (2008d) *NHS Next Stage Review: a vision for primary and community care*. London: Department of Health.

Department of Health (2009a) *Transforming Community Services and World Class Commissioning: resource pack for commissioners of community services*. London: Department of Health.

Department of Health (2009b) *Transforming Community Services: transformational guides*. www.dh.gov.uk/tcs (accessed 12 October 2010).

Department of Health (2009c) *Supporting People with Long Term Conditions: commissioning personalised care planning*. London: Department of Health.

Department of Health (2010) *Equity and Excellence: Liberating the NHS*. London: The Stationery Office.

Douglas V (2001) Living with a chronic leg ulcer: an insight into patients' experiences and feelings. *Journal of Wound Care* 9: 355–60.

Help The Aged (2007) *The Challenge of Dignity in Care – Upholding the Rights of the Individual*. London: Help the Aged.

Macleod R (2003) Setting the context: what do we mean by psycho-social care in palliative care? In: Lloyd-Williams M (ed) *Psychosocial Issues in Palliative Care* (2e). Oxford: Oxford University Press, pp.1–21.

Nuland SB (1993) *How We Die*. London: Chatto and Windus.

Nursing and Midwifery Council (2008) *Confidentiality*. London: Nursing and Midwifery Council. www.nmc-uk.org/Nurses-and-midwives/Advice-by-topic/A/Advice/Confidentiality/ (accessed 12 October 2010).

Persoon A, Heinen M, Van Der Vleuten C *et al* (2004) Leg ulcers: a review of their impact on daily life. *Journal of Clinical Nursing* 13: 341–54.

Posnett J, Franks P (2007) The costs of skin breakdown and ulceration in the UK. In: Smith and Nephew Foundation. *Skin Breakdown – The Silent Epidemic*. UK: SNFoundation.

Royal College of Nursing (2008) *Defending Dignity – Challenges and Opportunities for Nursing*. London: Royal College of Nursing.

Sturdy D (2007) Indignity in care: are you responsible? *Nursing Older People* 19(9): 9.

Walshe C (1995) Living with a venous leg ulcer: a descriptive study of patients' experiences. *Journal of Advanced Nursing* 22: 1092–100.

Webster C, Bryan K (2009) Older people's views on dignity and how it can be promoted in a hospital environment. *Journal of Clinical Nursing* 18: 1784–92.

CHAPTER 12

Dignity in acute and critical care

Lesley Baillie

INTRODUCTION

Patients are admitted for acute and critical care due to a wide range of health problems, including planned surgery, emergencies such as trauma, or acute problems associated with long-term health conditions. These admissions are often accompanied by anxiety, fear, loss of control and dependency. Patients in acute and critical care settings are also particularly vulnerable to diminished dignity due to the health conditions that led to their hospital admission, the associated procedures and care activities, and the nature of the care environment. Even someone who is usually fit and well and is admitted for planned surgery can be vulnerable to diminished dignity due to loss of control and temporary dependence. Patients who are admitted as emergencies face additional uncertainties and even less control over their situation. A relative in Douglas-Dunbar and Gardiner's (2007) study highlighted that going into hospital 'is one of the most vulnerable times of your life' (p.29).

Thus although staff working in these areas are often under immense pressure, they still need to deliver care with dignity. This chapter focuses on the dignity of adults undergoing acute and critical care and highlights the care activities, treatments, procedures and processes in these settings that may undermine dignity. The chapter will specifically consider how dignity can be promoted in accident and emergency (A&E) departments, intensive therapy units (ITUs), and during perioperative care.

LEARNING OUTCOMES

By the end of the chapter you will be able to:
➤ analyse the challenges to dignity in acute and critical care settings, including the vulnerability of patients and care environment issues
➤ explain how dignity can be promoted for patients undergoing acute and critical care in accident and emergency departments, intensive therapy units, and during perioperative care.

CHALLENGES TO DIGNITY IN ACUTE AND CRITICAL CARE SETTINGS

Changes in health and social care provision have led to the inpatient population being increasingly frail and with complex needs (Bridges *et al*, 2010) and thus many people who are admitted for acute and critical care are already vulnerable. Two-thirds of hospital beds in the UK are occupied by people aged over 65 years (Department of Health [DH], 2001) and one study found that 18% of patients attending A&E departments were older people (Downing and Wilson, 2005), many of whom may have complex and multiple needs, including cognitive impairment. The population of people with learning disabilities is increasing and living into older age, and they are very likely to need emergency care due to a high risk of acute health problems (Brown, 2005). Mencap's (2007) report detailed several acute hospital admissions of people with learning disabilities and highlighted many affronts to their dignity (*see* Chapter 14 for a detailed exploration of dignity for people with learning disabilities).

Patients admitted to acute hospitals follow a pathway through departments and wards, encountering numerous different staff and procedures along the way. Individual staff members therefore rarely see the patient's whole acute care experience, but in Box 12.1 I have related my mother's journey through acute and critical care. As you read this, reflect on the factors that might have affected her dignity, in relation to her health condition, the procedures she experienced, and the care environment factors.

Box 12.1 illustrates how a usually independent woman in control of her own life and health developed an acute illness leading to her emergency admission and rapidly increasing helplessness. On the orthopaedic ward she could do very little independently as she could not move, eat or carry out personal care without help. Many patients find it undignified to have to be assisted with personal care, and at one point my mother said to me: 'I have lost all my dignity now – there's none left'. Unusually for the UK, and because of her infection, she had the privacy of being in a side room; many other patients in acute care settings are cared for in multi-bed areas with privacy provided by curtains. In theatre and ITU, my mother was totally dependent on the healthcare team and technology to support her bodily functions. She was physically examined by various doctors, requiring bodily exposure, and she had necessary but invasive procedures including urinary catheterisation and intravenous cannulation. Box 12.1 highlights the vulnerability of patients admitted to acute and critical care. You will be able to relate this to many other patients who follow similar paths through acute and critical care services.

As well as caring for an increasingly vulnerable population of patients, staff in critical care settings deal with a rapid throughput of patients which includes transfer and admission at short notice and little time in which to build relationships. In my doctoral research based on a surgical ward (Baillie, 2007), several patients commented on the staff's excessive workload and most perceived

---

BOX 12.1 *An acute admission to hospital*

My mother was 72 years old, lived in her own house with her older husband and was usually independent. One Sunday evening, she was taken to the A&E department by ambulance on a stretcher after a home visit by her general practitioner. My mother had developed a severely swollen and painful knee and her doctor suspected an abscess. In A&E she was transferred onto a trolley. Her vital signs were recorded and oxygen administered as her oxygen saturation was low. She was examined by an orthopaedic doctor, blood samples were taken, she had an intravenous cannula inserted, intravenous fluids were started and she had an X-ray of her leg. She was admitted into a side room (due to her suspected infection) on an orthopaedic ward. Her leg remained painful and she had difficulty in moving. She was unable to pass urine and so a urethral catheter was inserted. The following day she was prepared for theatre and her abscess was drained under general anaesthetic. Over the next few days, despite intravenous antibiotics, her condition deteriorated. Following blood cultures, she was diagnosed with septicaemia. She became increasingly breathless and she could eat only very small amounts, which were given to her on a spoon. She had a bedbath each day and used a bedpan to empty her bowels. She was examined by the orthopaedic and medical teams regularly. On her 7th day of admission she returned to theatre for a further drainage of abscess, after which she developed respiratory failure in recovery. She remained in recovery for several hours while an ITU bed was made available so she could be ventilated. On the 4th day in ITU her active treatment was stopped as she was now in multi-organ failure. Her sedation was increased and she died, with us, her family, by her bedside.

(source: Lesley Baillie)

---

a resulting adverse effect on their dignity, mainly because staff could appear brusque or off-hand. For example, one patient in this study commented that due to workload, staff did not introduce themselves, as 'They haven't time to keep stopping to talk to people' (p.147). Another patient, who had had major surgery, expressed that the hospital's busy routine and associated paperwork took priority over what he termed the 'care aspect', which he associated with dignity:

> Because it's a busy hospital – you've got such a busy routine that's perpetually changing – there's so much emphasis on them doing their work and they will do that and the patient just happens to be there. Their work goes before the patient . . . they're so busy doing what they're doing, filling in their forms, doing everything in the way they have to do it. The care aspect – it's quite difficult to know whether the care aspect is really really there (Baillie, 2007, p.148).

Another patient considered that the high workload led to a lack of individuality, illustrating her view by explaining that when she arrived at theatre she had to wait outside on a stretcher for a long time as the anaesthetist was double booked:

> It just makes you aware that you are patient number nine hundred and fifty-nine and you don't matter. You're in a meat market. And you're on a conveyor belt (Baillie, 2007, p.147).

Nursing staff, too, recognised the impact that busyness had on dignity; one senior nurse said:

> I suppose if staff appear very busy then that can impact upon dignity . . . that's almost unavoidable as well. If people are busy then they are busy and we both know how difficult it is when you've got a bay with six beds in and you've got somebody dying in that bay and you've got somebody else who's getting better and going home and you're trying to deal with different people going through different experiences (Baillie, 2007, p.148).

Nevertheless, I observed some staff who were working under immense pressure on the ward and yet still promoted patients' dignity. Staff who work in acute and critical care settings need skills to rapidly build rapport with patients and relatives despite the busy workload. As Bridges *et al* (2010) highlighted, for older people undergoing acute care, relationships with staff have a crucial impact on their care experience. Furthermore, Douglas-Dunbar and Gardiner (2007) asserted the importance of hospital staff developing a therapeutic relationship with the carer as well as the person with dementia.

Acute and critical care settings generally use a lot of technical equipment, which may impact on caring (Randle, 2001; Picker Institute, 2008). In Douglas-Dunbar and Gardiner's (2007) study of relatives of people with dementia admitted to hospital, one carer expressed that while the technology used may be life saving, 'the treatment of the person as an individual has somehow been lost' (p.29).

However, in Alliex and Irurita's (2004) study, nurses described making additional efforts to meet patients' humanistic needs in the presence of technology, which they referred to as 'maximising', and which consisted of:

➤ *maintaining presence*: offering help, popping in, giving time. For example, A&E staff can pop in to cubicles and check whether patients need anything
➤ *minimising the impact of technology*: staff can use social interaction, including humour if appropriate, and understate the technology used rather than focusing on it
➤ *individualising interactions*: considering patients' likes, doing little things (for example, making a telephone call for a patient), portraying a caring demeanour and kindness.

In essence, technology should not pose a barrier to dignified care, as long as staff continue to focus on the patient as a human being rather than on the technology alone. In my own experience as a relative (Box 12.1), most ITU staff did convey compassion alongside efficient use of technology in my mother's care.

Overall, patient frailty and vulnerability, invasive treatments and care, rapid patient throughput and technology are all challenges to dignity in acute and critical care. Nevertheless, there is much that staff in these settings can do to promote the dignity of patients. Earlier chapters of this book considered in detail how the care environment (Chapter 5) and staff behaviour (Chapter 6) can promote dignity in care. These principles can all be applied to acute and critical care settings. The next sections of this chapter consider some specific aspects of how healthcare professionals can promote dignity in A&E departments, during perioperative care and in ITU settings.

PROMOTING DIGNITY IN ACCIDENT AND EMERGENCY DEPARTMENTS

The Healthcare Commission (HCC) (2008) reported that during 2007/2008, there were 19.1 million attendances at A&E departments and urgent care centres in England and most patients were positive about their experiences. However, the HCC (2008) expressed concern that the needs of patients with complex or particular individual needs (such as vulnerable adults, people with disabilities) were not always met and patients were not always treated with dignity and respect. The HCC (2008) pointed out that when patients have negative experiences in A&E, particularly if they feel they have not been treated with dignity, they will feel upset and anxious about using services in the future. Reflective activity 12.1 includes some reflective questions about dignity in A&E.

Byrne (1997) found that A&E nurses viewed their role as one that was predominantly concerned with providing urgent physical care. While they acknowledged that many people attending A&E would be anxious, one nurse expressed that when A&E is busy 'the "patient as a person" thing gets forgotten' (p.97). However, just treating patients' physical conditions, without treating them as human beings, can lead to a negative experience of the A&E department. Look at your answers to the reflective questions: did you feel you were treated as a

Reflective activity 12.1 Reflecting on A&E experiences

You will almost certainly have attended A&E at some stage as a patient or relative. Reflect on the following:

➤ how did you feel when you first arrived in A&E?
➤ what were your *first* impressions of the staff you met and the A&E environment? How did these affect the rest of your A&E visit?
➤ how did the A&E environment affect your dignity?
➤ how did the way staff behaved towards you affect your dignity?

human being in A&E? An A&E visit is a significant event for many people, as it occurs suddenly, is often accompanied by pain, fear, stress and anxiety, and patients have had no opportunity to prepare physically, socially or psychologically (Baillie, 2005). Ford *et al* (2008) pointed out that emergency care settings are often the 'front doors' through which many patients start their healthcare journeys, so it is very important that dignity begins there. At the 2007 Royal College of Nursing (RCN) Emergency Care Association annual conference, the Patients Association gave examples of staff behaviour that diminished dignity in emergency departments (Ford *et al*, 2008). As a result, the two organisations jointly developed a set of nine 'dignity principles' that patients accessing emergency care should expect (*see* Box 12.2). Adhering to the principles in Box 12.2 should help to ensure that patients feel comfortable, in control and valued, which is important for patients to feel that their dignity is promoted (Baillie, 2009). Here we will consider patients' A&E experiences in more detail and include further details about promoting dignity in this environment.

In the UK, there is currently a four-hour target for A&E departments: patients should have been assessed, treated and either discharged or admitted within four hours. The Healthcare Commission (2008) reported that 97.9% of patients in A&E departments and urgent care centres were dealt with within four hours. While a speedy journey through A&E is generally in patients' best interests, staff have a tight time frame during which they must help patients feel that they have been treated as individuals and cared for as human beings. Therefore, A&E staff need to be able to develop a rapport with patients rapidly, and furthermore:

> Nurses should aim to be kind and courteous and even in the hectic pace of an A&E department it should be possible to accompany physical care with pleasantries and friendliness which helps people feel that they matter (reprinted from Baillie, 2005, p.13, with permission from Elsevier).

BOX 12.2 *The nine emergency care dignity principles: what patients can expect*

1. The reception staff will be welcoming, courteous and helpful.
2. You will be given a rough estimate of how long you should expect to wait before being seen by a healthcare professional.
3. All healthcare professionals dealing directly with you will formally introduce themselves and their role.
4. All staff will ask you how you would like to be addressed, either formally, by using your title and surname, or more informally, by using your first or other preferred name.
5. You will be looked after in a clean and safe environment. All staff will wash or cleanse their hands regularly and before each patient contact.
6. You will be asked for your informed consent before any procedure is initiated.
7. You will be kept up to date with information about your treatment plan. Any information obtained will be recorded and remain strictly confidential. We may, however, need to share some information with other health and social care professionals. Please feel free to ask about this in more detail.
8. You will be treated with respect and dignity at all times.
9. Staff will do their best to respect and address any religious or cultural needs if you make them aware.

(RCN, 2008; used with kind permission from the Royal College of Nursing)

This statement is applicable to all staff dealing with A&E patients, such as radiographers and medical staff, as well as nurses. When meeting patients for the first time in an acute care situation, staff should adopt a non-judgmental approach, avoid stereotyping and portray an appropriate level of understanding and compassion for the person's situation (Bowman and Thompson, 1998). In A&E, this must be portrayed during an initial brief encounter where there is, correctly, a focus on identifying urgent needs.

Patients attend A&E departments for all sorts of reasons. Initially they are triaged and from there they are referred to the appropriate area of the department, which might be the minor injuries area, major area or resuscitation area. In the minor injuries area, staff should be courteous, keep patients informed and protect privacy during treatment. Patients treated in the minor injuries area may be upset due to the cause of injury (for example, dog bite, assault), anxious and in some discomfort. They may be concerned about the effect on their body image (for example, with facial injuries) or on their employment (for example, a self-employed carpenter with a hand injury). The approach of staff has a strong influence on the dignity of patients in these situations.

In the major area of A&E, the patient care pathway usually involves initial assessment and undressing for examination, followed by further investigations and treatment. Staff can do much to promote dignity through introducing themselves to patients and their relatives, addressing patients politely and by the name they prefer, explaining what will happen, keeping patients and their relatives informed, and ensuring that they have call bells, which gives some control. Relatives or friends who are accompanying patients should remain with them as much as possible, as long as this is the patient's wish. Douglas-Dunbar and Gardiner (2007) highlighted how vulnerable older carers can feel when their relative with dementia is admitted to hospital; they reported feeling ignored and not kept informed. While most patients will need to undress so that they can be properly examined and no important problem is missed, staff should approach this sensitively. They should explain why it is necessary to undress, and gain consent to proceed, leave underwear on unless there is a reason to remove it (for example, soiling), provide a gown to wear and linen to cover the patient, and put clothing carefully into a labelled bag. Staff should ensure that the patient knows where their belongings are and that they are safe, and put any soiled clothing into a separate bag. If it is not necessary to keep the patient nil by mouth, then staff should offer a drink. They should explain to patients who must remain nil by mouth (for example, swallowing problem, likelihood of emergency surgery) why they cannot have a drink, and offer mouthwashes for comfort.

Privacy should always be given during examinations and this is of paramount concern for intimate examinations (for example, vaginal or rectal). The RCN (2006) *Guidelines for Vaginal and Pelvic Examinations* advise the use of a warm private room with a lock on the door, that couches and trolleys should face away from the door, and that there should be toilets and bathrooms near the examination rooms. For women having miscarriages in the emergency department, Bryant (2008) suggested that all equipment needed should be available so staff do not have to leave the room during procedures, and that hygiene packs should be available containing pants, pads, wipes and disposal bags. Prior to examinations, staff should explicitly ask for consent to examine, and recheck consent during the procedure as necessary. A chaperone will be required during intimate examinations; chaperones should introduce themselves and stay where the patient can see them. If the examination is uncomfortable or distressing, the chaperone should offer a hand to hold and express concern and reassurance. Certain procedures need a team of staff; for example, a patient with a suspected cervical spine injury will need four staff to log-roll while the patient is examined, which will include checking for sensation down to the base of the spine. Dignity can be promoted by introductions, explanations and minimising exposure. Some A&E patients will be embarrassed by their appearance; they may have been incontinent, or not have bathed today or put on clean clothes. For some patients, having to have an intimate examination, use a bedpan or give a urine sample will be the first time they have experienced this in their lives. Therefore, staff dealing with A&E patients should be sensitive, reassuring and aware of cultural and religious needs too.

Patients treated in the resuscitation area of an emergency department are those who are most acutely unwell or unstable, for example, those with cardiac chest pain or major trauma. The priority is to assess them rapidly, and carry out urgent investigations and treatments. The team may have to quickly remove clothing, possibly by cutting, in order to examine and treat the patient. Staff should approach these urgent activities in a way that promotes dignity; it is still possible to give explanations and gain consent, keep patients' bodies covered most of the time and address patients' concerns. Resuscitation attempts can appear very undignified indeed, as cardiac compressions, airway management and defibrillation are all rapidly delivered. It is very important that, following the initial urgent activity, any dignity loss is quickly restored. When relatives are brought in to see patients following an unsuccessful resuscitation attempt, the patient's appearance may remain with them forever. It is paramount to spend some time tidying up the patient and the near environment, removing used equipment, washing away any blood, closing eyes and putting in dentures, wiping away blood, vomit, etc. from the face, putting a clean gown on the

---

BOX 12.3 *A relative's experience*

When we were taken to his bed we were not prepared for the horrific sight of seeing him, eyes wide open with a resuscitation tube down his throat. This image has traumatised not only us but also my sister and brother in law for the rest of our lives! When my daughter asked if the tube could be removed the nurse informed us that it had to stay for legal reasons. We should have been warned beforehand so that we could have made an informed choice of whether to see him or not. This haunting image of a proud man who looked as if he had starved to death will stay with us forever!

(Patients Association, 2009, pp.34–5, reprinted with permission from The Patients Association)

patient, spigoting any tubes attached, covering the patient with a blanket and putting a clean pillow under the patient's head. Airway equipment inserted during the resuscitation attempt may have to be left in for post mortem, as per hospital guidelines. It is important to explain to relatives, and significant others who wish to see the patient, exactly what to expect prior to visiting, thus enabling them to make an informed choice. Box 12.3 includes a relative's account which illustrates the consequences of a lack of preparation. A&E staff should aim to portray to relatives that the patient who has died suddenly has been treated with dignity and care, with recognition for the important human being that they are. Relatives should be treated with dignity; nursing and medical staff should display kindness and compassion and provide information in a non-hurried manner and give time for questions.

PROMOTING THE DIGNITY OF PATIENTS DURING PERIOPERATIVE CARE

Perioperative care has many potential effects on dignity; we will consider pre-operative care, dignity in the operating theatre, and immediate postoperative care.

Preoperative care

There are a number of ways in which preparation for theatre can impact on dignity; for example, Goldberg *et al* (2009) highlighted that marking surgical sites on patients' bodies, particularly in more intimate areas, can undermine dignity. Matiti and Sharman (1999) identified how traditional practice in preoperative care can threaten dignity as patients may be asked to remove their clothes, jewellery, cosmetics and dentures, all of which can be part of their identity. However, jewellery only really needs to be removed if it will interfere with the operation site, and jewellery that may come into contact with diathermy equipment can be covered with tape. Matiti and Sharman (1999) highlighted patients' discomfort about removing their dentures, for example: 'I was very, very embarrassed, as I cannot take my dentures out, even in front of my family'. However, securely fitted dentures do not actually need removing prior to surgery. Dentures that do need removal can be taken out in the anaesthetic room, put into a labelled pot and replaced as soon as the patient wakes up in recovery. Patients can be encouraged to wear disposable underwear to theatre. Hair removal can diminish dignity, especially hair on the head. Shaving can be avoided as much as possible; if skin is prepared with appropriate solution, procedures can often be carried out with no or minimal hair shaving.

Operation gowns have been found to threaten dignity as they can expose patients (Walsh and Kowanko, 2002; Woogara, 2005; Baillie, 2009). Therefore, ward staff should not ask patients to change into gowns earlier than necessary and patients who walk to theatre in gowns must have dressing gowns to wear. On arrival in theatre, patients enter the anaesthetic room. Here, staff should greet the patient and introduce themselves and explain what is going to happen. They should ask the patient how they would like to be addressed and record this so that the recovery room staff can use the patient's preferred name when waking them. While preparing to administer the anaesthetic, staff should be pleasant and conversational and not talk over the patient. The aim is for the patient to feel cared about and safe in the hands of the operating department staff.

Care during theatre

Marshall (1994) highlighted that anaesthetised patients entrust the theatre team with maintaining their dignity and safety. However, Chapter 8, Box 8.1 provides an example of a mother who, following caesarean section, was left exposed and ignored. She described her shame and embarrassment at being left exposed like 'a slab of meat'. Operating department staff should attend to privacy of the patient by avoiding any unnecessary exposure and not having extra observers present unless the patient gave permission. Some patients will be awake or sedated during the procedure (rather than unconscious) as they have local or epidural anaesthesia. Communication with these patients is absolutely crucial: politeness and courtesy, explanations and keeping patients informed along with a kind and caring approach.

Patients are often acutely aware that intimate areas of their bodies will be exposed and invaded in theatre. For example, a patient expressed embarrassment about having bladder surgery, saying:

> I mean in my case, I had an operation on the bladder so obviously the thought of what they were going to do to me was a feeling of – oh – how awful, you know (Baillie, 2007, p.166).

Her embarrassment led to her opting for a general anaesthetic, as undergoing surgery while she was awake during epidural anaesthesia would have been too 'humiliating' to contemplate.

Many other patients will have such procedures carried out while they are awake and operating staff should be sensitive and discreet and attend to privacy. Theatre staff should also ensure that they clean the patient thoroughly when surgery is completed, before transfer to recovery, so that they are not covered by dried blood or other body fluids and solutions.

Immediate postoperative care

Immediately postoperatively, in the recovery room and following transfer to the ward or unit, patients are in a very vulnerable situation. There is potential for them to be in pain or to vomit, though this should generally be controlled with medication. They are unable to move or do anything for themselves. In addition, they may be cared for in a multi-patient area with only curtains for privacy. Staff should ensure that patients' comfort, safety and dignity are promoted. They should ensure dentures are replaced (if applicable) and that, despite the many bodily attachments (drains, catheter, infusions) that may be present, patients' bodily privacy is maintained. Staff should address the patient by their preferred name while awakening them, give explanations and gently find out the cause of any apparent distress.

PROMOTING THE DIGNITY OF PATIENTS IN INTENSIVE THERAPY UNITS

Patients admitted to ITU are critically ill and totally dependent on the staff caring for them. While some patients are unconscious, others will be awake as they are being weaned from mechanical ventilation but they will be physically too weak to self-care. Holland *et al* (1997) interviewed patients about their recollections of their ITU stay; they stated that it was easier to cope with the stress of ITU if nurses treated them with respect and dignity. Several other studies have investigated perspectives of dignity for ITU patients. In the study of Plakas *et al* (2009), based in Greece, relatives of ITU patients considered that dignity related to cleanliness of the patient's body and respectful care of the patient, including relief of pain and suffering. Pokorny (1989) interviewed patients who had been in ITU for at least 24 hours following cardiovascular bypass surgery about their perceptions of their dignity while they were in ITU. The patients identified privacy, control, independence, competence and caring as attributes of dignity. Arguably, ITU patients and their relatives should be able to count on staff to be competent and caring, but control and independence could be more elusive. However, staff could consider how these attributes might apply, for example, by including and involving patients' relatives. Finding out from relatives about the patient, their likes and dislikes and how they like to be addressed can help staff to approach the patient as an individual. Engström and Söderberg (2004) found that partners of critically ill spouses felt secure when they were kept informed. They also considered it important that staff showed respect for the critically ill person and acted as if they were conscious and could hear everything. One patient's partner said that the nurses were good 'acting as if my husband was conscious' but that one of the doctors 'was the only one who didn't' (p.302). She said that he had stood smiling, making a long speech, which she thought was 'terrible'.

Challenges to the privacy of patients in ITU relate to both the care environment and the nature of patients' conditions. In ITU, patients are likely to be cared for in bays with screens used for privacy, and they have multiple attachments to their bodies, for treatment and monitoring purposes. Thus, Turnock and Kelleher (2001) asserted that it is common practice in ITU for patients to be nursed naked (though covered with linen), for the convenience of clinical procedures such as patient observation or integrity of invasive equipment. They further suggested that minimising exposure of genitalia can be problematic due to the invasive equipment attached and that the clinical team require great skills to prevent patient exposure. Other factors highlighted were reduced patient consciousness, and the need to perform many tasks rapidly to avoid compromising a physiologically unstable patient. Turnock and Kelleher (2001) found that most exposure occurred during clinical procedures, in particular, technical procedures and repositioning. Some staff demonstrated a lack of awareness for unconscious patients' dignity by saying, of the impact of bodily exposure on patients and their relatives: 'If the patients can't be asked, they can't get stressed by it'. However, one nurse acknowledged the impact on relatives and another nurse recognised that failing to cover patients up could lead to dehumanisation. Turnock and Kelleher (2001) identified that exposure could be reduced by staff being more vigilant about clothing and screening patients, thoroughly preparing the bed area and removing unnecessary equipment, encouraging staff to ask permission before entering bed curtains, and assessing patients' privacy and dignity needs by involving relatives. Thus, although it may be more challenging to promote privacy in ITU, it is still possible, with care and thoughtfulness.

A certain number of patients in ITU, like my mother (*see* Box 12.1), will deteriorate and die. Chapter 10 explores dignity at the end of life in detail, and much of this discussion is relevant in ITU as well. However, in ITU, dying has added complexity; the major focus is on reviving and saving so once the care focus changes to de-escalation of treatment and allowing the dying process, some staff may view the situation as failure. Nevertheless, critical care nurses have expressed that facilitating dying with dignity is important in end-of-life-care (Kirchhoff *et al*, 2000; Beckstrand *et al*, 2006; Plakas *et al*, 2009). Beckstrand *et al* (2006) suggested that facilitators to providing a good death include encouraging family members to stay with the patient, providing facilities for the family, soothing music, quiet places for prayer and meditation and family gatherings. However, not all ITUs will have ideal facilities for relatives, and privacy for the patient and family can be difficult as many patients will be in a screened bay, outside which the busy unit's work continues. ITU staff can, nevertheless, do much to promote dignity through their communication with patients and their relatives and attending to comfort and fundamental care.

CONCLUSION

In acute and critical care settings, patients are particularly vulnerable to a loss of dignity due to their health status and the treatments needed. The care environment can be depersonalising and unwelcoming to patients and their relatives. Staff working in these settings are often under considerable pressure and are dealing with groups of acutely unwell patients, in sometimes less than ideal environments. However, as dignity is very important to acute and critical care patients, staff must attend to privacy, ensure treatments and care are performed competently and confidently to a high standard, and that they communicate with patients and their relatives in a way that helps them to feel comfortable, in control and valued. The care environment plays an important role in supporting staff to promote dignity and should have the facilities to enable privacy and high-quality care. Acutely unwell patients who feel that their dignity is preserved by staff caring for them can concentrate on their recovery and feel confident in those they are dependent on.

ACKNOWLEDGEMENTS

I would like to thank Jessica Baillie, Lorraine Ilott, Sue Maddex and Ibraheim Almakari for their comments and suggestions during the preparation of this chapter.

REFERENCES

Alliex S, Irurita VF (2004) Caring in a technological environment: how is this possible? *Contemporary Nurse* 17(1–2): 32–43.

Baillie L (2005) An exploration of nurse-patient relationships in Accident and Emergency. *Accident and Emergency Nursing* 13(1): 9–14.

Baillie L (2007) *Patient Dignity in an Acute Hospital Setting* Unpublished thesis. London: South Bank University.

Baillie L (2009) Patient dignity in an acute hospital setting: a case study. *International Journal of Nursing Studies* 46: 22–36.

Beckstrand RL, Callister LC, Kirchhoff KT (2006) Providing a 'good death': critical care nurses' suggestions for improving end-of-life care. *American Journal of Critical Care* 15(1): 38–45.

Bowman GS, Thompson DR (1998) Therapeutic nursing in acute care. In: McMahon R, Pearson A (eds) *Nursing as Therapy* (2e). Cheltenham: Stanley Thornes.

Bridges J, Flatley M, Meyer J (2010) Older people's and relatives' experiences in acute care settings: systematic review and synthesis of qualitative studies. *International Journal of Nursing Studies* 47: 89–107.

Brown M (2005) Emergency care for people with learning disabilities: what all nurses and midwives need to know. *Accident and Emergency Nursing* 13: 224–31.

Bryant H (2008) Maintaining patient dignity and offering support after miscarriage. *Emergency Nurse* 15(9): 26–9.

Byrne G (1997) Understanding nurses' communication with patients in accident and emergency departments using a symbolic interactionist perspective. *Journal of Advanced Nursing* 26(1): 93–100.

Department of Health (2001) *The National Service Framework for Older People.* London: Department of Health.

Douglas-Dunbar M, Gardiner P (2007) Support for carers of people with dementia during hospital admissions. *Nursing Older People* **16**(5): 810–18.

Downing A, Wilson R (2005) Older people's use of Accident and Emergency services. *Age and Ageing* **34**: 24–30.

Engström Ä, Söderberg S (2004) The experiences of partners of critically ill persons in an intensive care unit. *Intensive and Critical Care Nursing* **20**: 299–308.

Ford P, Hayward M, Baillie L *et al* (2008) Sticking to our principles. *Emergency Nurse* **16**(4): 4–5.

Goldberg AE, Harnish JL, Stegienko S, Urbach DR (2009) Attitudes of patients and care providers toward a surgical site marking policy. *Surgical Innovation* **16**: 249–57.

Healthcare Commission (2008) *Not Just a Matter of Time: a review of urgent and emergency care services in England.* London: Healthcare Commission.

Holland C, Cason CL, Prater LR (1997) Patients' recollections of critical care. *Dimensions of Critical Care Nursing* **16**(3): 132–41.

Kirchhoff KT, Spuhler V, Walker L *et al* (2000) Intensive care nurses' experiences with end-of-life care. *American Journal of Critical Care* **9**(1): 36–42.

Marshall C (1994) The concept of advocacy. *British Journal of Theatre Nursing* **4**(2): 11–13.

Matiti MR, Sharman J (1999) Dignity: a study of preoperative patients. *Nursing Standard* **14**(13): 32–5.

Mencap (2007) *Death by Indifference.* London: Mencap.

Patients Association (2009) *Patients . . . Not Numbers, People . . . Not Statistics.* London: Patients Association.

Picker Institute (2008) *The Challenge of Assessing Dignity in Care.* London: Help the Aged.

Plakas S, Cant B, Taket A (2009) The experiences of critically ill patients in Greece: a social constructionist grounded theory study. *Intensive and Critical Care Nursing* **25**: 10–20.

Pokorny ME (1989) *The Effect of Nursing Care on Human Dignity in the Critically Ill Adult.* Unpublished PhD thesis. University of Virginia.

Randle J (2001) Past caring? The influence of technology. *Nurse Education Today* **1**: 157–65.

Royal College of Nursing (2006) *Guidelines for Vaginal and Pelvic Examinations.* London: Royal College of Nursing.

Royal College of Nursing (2008) *Dignity A&E poster.* London: Royal College of Nursing.

Turnock C, Kelleher M (2001) Maintaining patient dignity in intensive care settings. *Intensive and Critical Care Nursing* **17**(3): 144–54.

Walsh K, Kowanko I (2002) Nurses' and patients' perceptions of dignity. *International Journal of Nursing Practice* **8**(3): 143–51.

Woogara J (2005) Patients' privacy of the person and human rights. *Nursing Ethics* **12**(3): 273–87.

CHAPTER 13

Dignity in mental health: listening to the flying saint

Gemma Stacey and Theodore Stickley

INTRODUCTION

Research exploring the views of people who use mental health services has found people often feel stripped of dignity in the mental health system, even though the maintenance of dignity is recognised as crucial to recovery from mental health problems. This chapter explores the key areas identified within recent policy and research, which require substantial attention if practitioners are to maintain the dignity of people who use mental health services. We aim to expose the constraints of the current mental health system that contribute to the lack of dignified care reported by service users and carers. The dilemmas which face mental health practitioners will be critically discussed in light of the impact of mental health law and professional ethics surrounding this issue.

We hope that this chapter will enable you to understand the importance of promoting dignified care by relating theoretical concepts and discussions of dignity to practical examples. You will be encouraged to critically reflect upon the influence of public and practitioners' attitudes towards people who use mental health services in all healthcare settings. This will enable you to consider ways in which you can contribute to providing dignified care, and in doing so challenge the stigma and discrimination towards people who use mental health services, which is prevalent not only amongst wider society, but also within healthcare itself.

LEARNING OUTCOMES

By the end of this chapter you will be able to:
➤ discuss the position of dignity in mental healthcare and its relationship with the concept of recovery
➤ critically consider the underlying issues that present barriers to maintaining dignity within mental healthcare
➤ explore the significance of values when promoting dignified mental healthcare

➤ identify the issues within specific mental healthcare settings where provision of dignified care is most at risk

➤ apply these discussions to practice-based scenarios to consider how to promote dignity in practice.

A BRIEF HISTORY OF MENTAL HEALTHCARE

Before we begin to consider dignity in mental healthcare, it is important to give a brief historical background of the development of mental health services in the United Kingdom (UK). This will allow you to see the origins of current approaches to working with people who have been diagnosed with mental health problems and consider how these historical influences impact on the way people are viewed and treated in society today.

Treatment in mental health has had a chequered history. In fact, while medical care might have its origins in ancient Greece, mental healthcare only dates back to the Enlightenment era (the 'Age of Reason'). It was during this period that in Europe, social care became formalised and institutional solutions were offered to people who were considered 'mad'. These people were often referred to as 'lunatics'. Madhouses and lunatic asylums therefore came into existence. Before this development, those considered mad were often left to fend for themselves, and were cared for by families and communities or religious institutions. Around the 1790s, humane methods of treatment were being developed in institutions and this became known as 'moral treatment of the mentally ill'. In the Victorian period, large institutions were built, many of which exist to this day, although virtually all of the people who lived within these settings have long since been discharged into the community.

What became established during this fairly recent era, however, was the recognition that 'madness' or 'lunacy' was in fact a medical condition. This apparent progression in thinking coincided with the rise of the medical profession and it was at this point in history that 'madness' became medicalised. As such, mental illnesses had symptoms; these symptoms could be interpreted by a medical practitioner as symptoms of a recognisable illness. Thus, the illness could be diagnosed and a treatment could be prescribed. While on the one hand this significant development was seen as scientific progress, on the other hand people's social, psychological and emotional experiences came to be regarded as 'illness'. Therefore, people often received treatment inappropriately. Sometimes these treatments were later considered barbaric. For example, people were admitted to asylums for reasons we would now consider extraordinary, such as being pregnant outside wedlock, for having religious experiences, for being homosexual. Treatments included mechanical restraints, straitjackets, muzzles and so on. In the last century, insulin shock therapy was introduced, as well as electroconvulsive therapy, which is still used today.

Thousands of people had parts of their brains removed through a procedure called 'lobotomy'. At the time, these treatments were not generally considered barbaric; rather, they were implemented because they were based upon the best evidence of the day.

In the middle of the last century, more efficient drugs were developed which, some would argue, have effectively restrained people through chemicals rather than through chains and locks. Furthermore, although hospital wards were unlocked from the 1960s onwards, they have quite recently become locked once again in the UK under the era of New Labour (van der Merwe *et al*, 2009). Drug treatments have improved enormously, enabling people to lead seemingly normal lives, although the side-effects of psychotropic medication are themselves devastating for some people.

The effect of both the confinement of the mentally ill and subsequent seemingly punishing treatments was that people with a mental illness diagnosis became deeply stigmatised in society. The asylums became feared and threatening institutions. People who were treated in them became social pariahs. While we may like to think we live in more enlightened times, research evidence suggests that this social stigma is as strong today as it ever was. For a more detailed account of the history of mental health services and its relationship with nursing, please see Nolan (1999).

Complex mental health laws have been developed that enforce treatment for some people diagnosed as mentally ill who are considered to be a danger to themselves or to the public. The implementation of the Mental Health Act (1983), amended by the Mental Health Act 2007, falls upon mental healthcare workers and is fraught with complexity. It is hard to argue against mental health law that seeks to protect individuals and society from harm. However, the issues are not straightforward. Often, people are sectioned under mental health law and detained in hospital because there are no other alternatives. Issues of dignity in mental healthcare therefore may relate to legal issues such as human rights. Later in this chapter we offer two scenarios that illustrate the complexities in maintaining dignity in mental healthcare.

THE POSITION OF DIGNITY IN MENTAL HEALTHCARE

The following section of this chapter identifies the current mental health policy, which supports the need for improvements in the provision of dignified care as part of the recovery and social inclusion agenda. It explores the research evidence which has contributed to this political recognition by considering the issues of service user and carer experiences of using mental health services, public and professional attitudes towards this client group and the impact of stigma and discrimination on maintaining dignity.

The concept of recovery in mental healthcare

Contemporary mental health policy has identified recovery as a priority and it is currently positioned at the heart of its agenda. When related to mental health, the term 'recovery' has a slightly different meaning. It does not necessarily refer to a cure or restoration to the person's previous state of health. This is due to the recognition that people can and do live meaningful and fulfilling lives despite their mental health problems. The recovery movement was originally initiated by people who used mental health services, as many began to reject the labels and limitations that were placed upon them by mental health services and society. People began to tell their story of surviving the mental healthcare system and regaining a sense of self following many years of being exposed to dehumanising practices and undignified care. An excellent anthology illustrating such stories can be found in Barker *et al* (1999). The UK government began to incorporate concepts associated with recovery into policy in 1999 with the *National Service Framework* (NSF) *for Mental Health* (Department of Health [DH], 1999). This document identified that health and social care professionals should contribute to challenging the stigma and discrimination directed towards people with mental health problems and promote their social inclusion. To see examples of how this might be achieved through mental health promotion strategies, you should now complete Reflective activity 13.1.

Reflective activity 13.1 Investigate some mental health promotion strategies

Look up some examples of mental health promotion strategies that are using the media in a positive way by accessing the following:

➤ Shift: www.shift.org.uk/
➤ Time to Change: www.time-to-change.org.uk/
➤ BBC Headroom: www.bbc.co.uk/headroom/

This *National Service Framework for Mental Health* placed mental health promotion as a high priority for service providers which is certainly justified, as recent research exploring public attitudes towards people who use mental health services in England has found that negative attitudes have increased (Rethink, 2006; DH, 2008). The association between mental health problems and violence has worsened, and in a recent study, only 65% of respondents believed that people with mental health problems should be entitled to the same job opportunities as anyone else (TNS for Shift, CSIP, 2007). These findings are supported elsewhere. For example, in a study carried out by a mental health charity, 84% of people who use mental health services reported problems in gaining employment, accessing healthcare, and establishing relationships (Mind, 2004), and 49% have been harassed or physically attacked (Read and Barker, 1996).

With regard to dignity, the effects that stigma and subsequent discrimination may have on the individual cannot be emphasised enough. People who are diagnosed with a mental health problem often report experiencing a downward spiral of loss, social disadvantage and isolation. These experiences are regularly attributed to the media portrayal of people who use mental health services; however, some service users feel that it is also a consequence of the way people are treated in health services (Campbell, 1999). Tackling the stigma and subsequent discrimination attached to mental health problems must be a key role for the mental health worker if they are to promote recovery, and providing dignified care is an essential aspect of this. While there have been a number of high-profile campaigns in recent years (*see* Reflective activity 13.1), these are no substitute for the necessary grass-roots day-to-day work of tackling stigma and discrimination that workers and carers need to do among the people they come in contact with. If this is hard to imagine, you might like to consider how racial prejudice has been confronted in our society. While we are not asserting that this has been eliminated, it is much better than it was, say, 50 years ago. But this change has only come about by people standing up for what they believe in and fighting and arguing for social justice (Sayce, 2000). If this example is hard to relate to, you might also like to think about rights for women over the last 100 years or the rights of people described as lesbian or gay. We have a long way to go before we can say that people with mental health problems enjoy these same rights and protection in law. This is one reason why we discussed the law earlier, because it could be argued that the mental health law reinforces negative stereotypes because it emphasises danger and risk.

The *National Service Framework for Mental Health* (DH, 1999) also recognised that contemporary community mental health services should be organised in a way that would enable people who experience mental health problems to be cared for during periods of crisis in the least restrictive environment. This hoped to reduce the 'revolving door' scenario where people's lives were continuously disrupted, sometimes beyond repair, by frequent hospital admissions. This has resulted in the development of a model of community mental health services that can respond quickly to crisis and provide intensive treatment in the person's home environment in order to prevent or facilitate shorter admission to hospital. It is hoped that by enabling people to maintain their roles and relationships, the downward spiral of loss, which has previously been observed, can be challenged.

A number of other policy documents have continued to emphasise the importance of undoing the legacy of the large institutions and the stigma inherited from them (for example, *Modernising Mental Health Services*: DH, 1998; *The NHS Plan*: DH, 2000a). These documents include instructions for creating safe, sound, supportive services that should meet the needs of those who use them, and ways of involving and including people with mental health problems as equal citizens in society. The directives that have arisen from these documents are summarised in the first policy document directly advocating the recovery approach in mental healthcare, *The Journey to Recovery* (DH 2001a), which aims to inform all service providers of the significant shifts required in order to modernise mental healthcare.

The role of values

The directives outlined in the *National Service Framework for Mental Health* were supported by the publication of *The Ten Essential Shared Capabilities* (National Institute for Mental Health in England, 2004), which was developed in consultation with service users, carers and practitioners to provide a training and development framework for the mental healthcare workforce. It was acknowledged that previous frameworks did not go far enough in emphasising the influence of the values of practitioners in relation to the care they deliver or the importance of working in collaboration with service users and carers to focus on their strengths and challenge inequalities. This document makes specific reference to dignity in relation to respecting the diversity of people who use mental health services and promoting their right to make informed choices and for staff to take therapeutic risks. Some have referred to this as a 'dignity of risk' (Parsons, 2008). It recognised that a shift is required in the attitudes and values of practitioners if they are to genuinely facilitate recovery and give choice and control back to people who use mental health services.

The Chief Nursing Officer's review of mental health nursing (DH, 2006) also provides some valuable recommendations for mental health practice across the professions. This document is named *From Values to Action* and reiterates the principles of the essential shared capabilities. It identifies that dignity should be upheld by respecting the values of people who use mental health services through creating forums for shared decision making. The review recognises that this will sometimes involve advocating for vulnerable individuals who may not have a voice or may feel unable to assert their perspective. It also adds that the physical health of people who use mental health services has been severely neglected. It is proposed that their right to receive healthcare provision is often hindered by lack of recognition by mental health professionals and lack of access due to dismissive and stigmatising attitudes among general healthcare professionals.

Underpinning each of these policy documents and their successful implementation is the significance of the values and attitudes that the practitioner holds towards those with whom they are working. These initiatives are supported by the Values Based Practice agenda, which recognises that the decisions we make and the way we care for people are influenced not only by evidence, but also by what we believe is morally and ethically right (Woodbridge and Fullford, 2005). It is here where we can see how the issue of dignity is central to our actions. In order to explore the values you bring to your practice, you should now complete Reflective activity 13.2.

Reflective activity 13.2 Writing a professional philosophy statement

A professional philosophy is a personal statement that describes your own values, beliefs and theories about how nurses and midwives should practise and care for people who use health services. There is not necessarily a 'right' or 'wrong' way to write your statement. However, there are certain issues that you should probably consider when making the connections between what you believe about practice, how you practise and how you evaluate your practice.

Most simply, you can start by asking yourself:

➤ What are health services for?
➤ What do you think people who use health services should expect from care?
➤ What are your values, attitudes and beliefs about people who use health services?
➤ So, what approaches do you use that reflect this position (perhaps with a couple of examples)?

Now that you have written your professional philosophy statement, use a highlighter to identify which parts are influenced by your values.

How do you think this relates to providing dignified care?

DIGNITY IN SPECIFIC MENTAL HEALTH SETTINGS

The Dignity in Care campaign in England was launched in 2006 (*see* Chapter 4) and aims to eliminate tolerance of services that do not respect dignity (DH, 2009). This campaign has now been extended from older adults' services to include mental health services. The campaign has highlighted the key areas where maintaining dignity is at risk, one of which includes tackling stigma. Additionally, the campaign also prioritises older people's mental health and acute inpatient care. The campaign utilises dignity champions who are volunteers and work to increase the profile of dignity in practice areas. You can find out more about the Dignity in Care campaign by completing Reflective activity 13.3. This will give you the opportunity to see some examples of where dignity has been addressed in mental healthcare, for example, advocating working in partnership with people who use mental health services to achieve their goals to improve quality of life.

Reflective activity 13.3 Find out more about Dignity in Care within mental health

➤ Follow the link provided: www.dhcarenetworks.org.uk/dignityincare/index.cfm
➤ Read about some of the 'ideas from practice'
➤ What are your thoughts about these initiatives?

Older adults' mental healthcare

Chapter 9 discusses dignity in the context of older adults; however, a significant area of concern regarding the provision of dignified care arises from research exploring older people's experiences of using mental health services. Some older people might be considered the most vulnerable in society. This vulnerability might be multiplied if the person has experienced years of mental health problems, subsequent treatments and the social consequences. Furthermore, many thousands of people also become mentally unwell through dementia and Alzheimer's disease. When physical frailty is accompanied with mental frailty, the individual's dignity is at greatest risk.

The *National Service Framework for Older People* (DH, 2001b) emphasises the need for person-centred care. If care that is delivered to older people with mental health problems is truly person centred, then their dignity would be protected. However, there are multiple factors that jeopardise people's dignity in practice. As a principle, one key way to preserve the dignity of older people is to ensure that the views and wishes of service users or their carers are elicited and acted upon in meaningful ways. We would assert that this is the first key to ensuring dignity among this client group. A great deal more importance needs to be placed upon the needs of older people, especially those with mental health problems. This will become a considerably growing issue as the retired population increases. As with all areas of mental health, workers need to campaign for the needs of our clients and ensure that they receive the same rights and privileges as others in our society.

Stories are all too frequently told of abuse of older people in institutional care (Penhale, 2008). Significant improvements may only take place when individual workers demand the kind of quality of care at grass-roots level that is called for at policy level (DH, 2001b). Another area of concern is when older people with mental health needs are admitted to acute general health wards for physical conditions. Often, their mental health needs are not understood or catered for, perhaps because of the lack of understanding of mental health needs among general nurses. Obviously, this calls for greater education for inpatient staff and increased practice development in physical healthcare wards.

Inpatient mental healthcare

Our final area to consider, when thinking about the importance of dignity within mental healthcare, is the issues that arise for people who are admitted to inpatient units during periods of crisis. The Sainsbury Centre for Mental Health (SCMH) has identified from its research that the top priority for mental health service users is the improvement of conditions on inpatient units (SCMH, 2004). The research evidence suggests that people feel they are treated with far less dignity in these settings than in physical healthcare settings (SCMH, 1998, 2002, 2004), which is clearly a cause for concern. To illustrate the seriousness of these concerns, consider the following: in 2009, the NHS was criticised for the four unnecessary deaths a day among those in psychiatric inpatient care (Campbell, 2009). The National Patient Safety Agency (NPSA) reports that 1282 people in England died in what it calls 'patient safety incidents in mental health settings' in the period 2007–2008 (this is helpfully collated by Campbell, 2009). The figures include people who committed suicide, and those who died through violent incidents, medication safety errors and accidents, although it is unclear how many deaths were in each category.

Acute inpatient mental health services in the UK have been considered dysfunctional, failing (Dodds and Bowles, 2001), and denying individuals their human rights (SCMH, 2002). Staff morale is low and recruitment, retention and sickness are problematic. These problems are recognised by the DH (2002) and there are moves to improve care.

The mental health charity Mind (2004) has reported similar findings: only one in five of the respondents to their survey on acute wards felt that they were treated by staff with respect and dignity. Almost the same proportion (17%) stated that they were never treated by staff with respect and dignity. In its 13th biennial report 2007–2009, the Mental Health Act Commission (2009) has authoritatively addressed dignity in mental healthcare. It gives many examples of how this can be compromised, including absence of appropriate bedding and dirty linen. Restraint procedures are a common complaint in mental healthcare. The report gives an example of how undignified restraint can become, as people reported being restrained for lengthy periods in full view of others on the ward. It was identified that the absence of a seclusion room means that people may be restrained in the main ward area until they are considered calm enough to be released. It is recognised that this is clearly upsetting not only for the restrained person but also for those witnessing the restraint. There are examples in the literature that call for a positive focus on promoting dignity in physical restraint (Moylan, 2009).

Not all is bad, and blame should not rest with the nurses who work at grass-roots level with resource problems and low morale. The problems on acute wards are systemic. Answers to problems will only be found by looking at the bigger picture, incorporating philosophy, research, theory, practice and, most importantly, what service users say. However, for mental health workers to maintain the dignity of the individual on acute wards is exceptionally difficult.

There has been much research into service users' views of inpatient care, and familiar themes emerge:

➤ overuse of medication
➤ lack of therapy – counselling
➤ lack of therapeutic activities
➤ not socially inclusive
➤ poor environment
➤ poor resources
➤ frightening atmosphere (especially for women)
➤ lack of goals of the service
➤ inadequate evidence base for treatments
➤ lack of information
➤ lack of involvement and choice
➤ not person-centred care, little regard for background and culture
➤ African-Caribbean people overrepresented and more likely to be sectioned
➤ disconnection from community workers when inpatient
➤ staffing problems: low morale, lack of support, overuse of agency staff, inadequate training
➤ boredom (SCMH, 2002).

Very recently, there has also been an emphasis upon the negative effects of mixed-sex wards. The dangers posed to women, highlighted in the NPSA report (2006), showed that over 100 women were raped, sexually assaulted or sexually harassed in NHS mental health units over a two-year period monitored in this research. Almost three years after these findings have been made public, the issue of keeping vulnerable women safe while detained under section is still a long way from being resolved.

Specific recommendations have been made by the government in relation to mixed-sex accommodation on wards. In *Modernising Mental Health Services* (DH, 1998), the government outlined a strategy that aimed to ensure that people who were admitted to wards were protected from physical, psychological or sexual harm, as a means of providing dignified care. This document drew attention to the ward environment and attempted to enforce the eradication of any mixed-sex accommodation. However, a further operational policy was later published named *Safety, Privacy and Dignity in Mental Health Units*, which lowered expectations to single-sex sleeping accommodation and washing facilities (DH, 2000b). This is despite the recognition that a number of people admitted to these practice areas may have a history of being abused and may not feel safe mixing with the opposite sex. Furthermore, during periods of crisis some people's distress may lead to violent or abusive behaviour and therefore place people who are vulnerable at risk. This document also identifies the importance of assessment, in order to judge if a person is vulnerable to being abused or may abuse others. Additionally, the significance of fully investigating accusations of abuse is emphasised.

THINKING ABOUT DIGNITY IN MENTAL HEALTHCARE

In summary, the policy documents, research evidence and discussion outlined here identify several areas where dignity is central to providing recovery-orientated care. These include:

➤ challenging stigma and discrimination
➤ promoting social inclusion
➤ respecting diversity
➤ advocating for the individual's right to make choices and take risks
➤ facilitating shared decision making
➤ challenging disempowering practices
➤ promoting awareness of physical health issues
➤ providing safe care environments
➤ thinking about people holistically, not just medically.

In this chapter we have only introduced some of the complex ways to think about dignity in mental healthcare. The truth is, we could write a whole book on the subject. We want to emphasise that issues of dignity in mental healthcare are complex. With this in mind, we have included some complex scenarios for you to consider. Having said they are complex, they are based upon the authors' experiences in mental health settings and unfortunately are quite typical of situations that may arise in mental health work. Take a look at the scenarios in Reflective activities 13.4 and 13.5. Each scenario is followed by some critical questions. Please take time to think about these questions and have a go at answering them. By doing so, you will be addressing some of the complex questions workers need to grapple with when thinking about dignity in mental healthcare. Pseudonyms have been used in these exercises.

CONCLUSION

The material presented in this chapter is only a brief introduction to some of the issues that illustrate how dignity threads through all aspects of recovery-

Reflective activity 13.4 Maintaining dignified care in complex situations

Case study: Bernie

Bernie is a 24-year-old West Indian man living on his own in a small flat in a poor inner-city area. His neighbours have complained to the police that he has been playing loud music through the night. Bernie is a very big gentleman, and some of his (white) neighbours are frightened of him. Bernie is known to smoke cannabis. When the police arrived to investigate the situation, Bernie was shouting out of his window that he was the true king of Jamaica and was able to walk on water. When they discovered he had previous contact with social services, and a history of violent offences, the police arranged for a Mental Health Act assessment. When the doctors and the approved mental health practitioner (AMHP) arrived to assess him, Bernie refused to open his door. In preparation for the assessment, the AMHP had obtained a warrant to enter Bernie's premises by force if required. The riot police were called to break down the door and an ambulance was called to transport Bernie to hospital if required. A small group of Bernie's neighbours gathered around his flat to watch the proceedings. As the police broke down the door to Bernie's flat, they entered using CS gas and restrained him by force before leading him to the ambulance in handcuffs.

Critical questions
➤ How was Bernie's dignity compromised?
➤ How might some of this have been avoided?
➤ What might be the social consequences for Bernie following this incident?
➤ Imagine the effect of this incident on Bernie: how might he respond and how might he feel in the future about this incident?
➤ How would you feel if you were Bernie?
➤ Imagine the role of the nurses on the ward when Bernie is admitted: what problems might they face both immediately and in the days to follow?
➤ How might this incident affect Bernie's future?
➤ What might be some of the social influences related to this story?
➤ What might be some of the psychological influences related to this story?

Reflective activity 13.5 Maintaining dignified care in complex situations

Case Study: Imogen

Imogen is 17 years old. Her parents are both successful, well-educated professional people. She is an only child, and her parents have been told that she is predicted to achieve four grade As in her A-level exams. They are hoping she will be successful in gaining a place at Oxford University. Under the strain of her studies and the pressure she has felt from her parents, Imogen has been admitted to an assessment ward, having experienced what had been described as a 'mental breakdown'. Imogen prefers to dance around the ward naked claiming that she is Saint Catherine de Vigni, and she prefers to fly rather than walk. Her parents are clearly embarrassed by her behaviour as it started at home and she had previously paraded around the village wearing nothing more than a silk scarf.

Critical questions
➤ How was Imogen's dignity compromised?
➤ How might these incidents have been avoided?
➤ What might be the social consequences for Imogen following these incidents?
➤ Imagine the effect of these incidents on Imogen: how might she respond and how might she feel in the future about these incidents?
➤ How would you feel if you were Imogen?
➤ Imagine the role of the nurses on the ward with Imogen. What problems might they face both immediately and in the days to follow?
➤ How might these incidents affect Imogen's future?
➤ What might be some of the social influences related to this story?
➤ What might be some of the psychological influences related to this story?

orientated mental healthcare. As you can see, the issues are complex and there are many barriers to making dignified mental healthcare a reality in practice. However, if the fundamental values that inform our work are underpinned by a belief in the person's rights to equality and inclusion, dignified care will follow despite these barriers. Small shifts in the way we communicate choice to people who use mental health services and challenge disempowering practices will, and do, make a significant difference to individuals and families.

The European Parliament (2006), in its Green Paper entitled *Improving the Mental Health of the Population: a Strategy for the European Union*, calls for all people with mental health problems to be treated with dignity and humanity and for them to have their human rights upheld by healthcare professionals. Excellent examples of dignified approaches to mental healthcare are reported in the literature, which remind us that barriers are challenges that can be overcome; however, there is still much more to be done in order to say that we have succeeded in providing wholly dignified mental healthcare.

REFERENCES

Barker P, Campbell P, Davidson B (1999) *From the Ashes of Experience: reflections on madness, survival and growth*. London: Whurr.

Campbell D (2009) Four psychiatric patients dying each day in NHS care. *Observer* 12 April.

Campbell P (1999) The service user/survivor movement. In: Newnes C, Holmes G, Dunn C (eds) *This is Madness: a critical look at psychiatry and the future of mental health services*. Ross-on-Wye: PCCS Books, pp.195–210.

Department of Health (1998) *Modernising Mental Health Services*. London: Department of Health.

Department of Health (1999) *The National Service Framework for Mental Health*. London: Department of Health.

Department of Health (2000a) *The NHS Plan*. London: Department of Health.

Department of Health (2000b) *Safety, Privacy and Dignity in Mental Health Units: guidance on mixed sex accommodation for mental health services*. London: Department of Health.

Department of Health (2001a) *The Journey to Recovery*. London: Department of Health.

Department of Health (2001b) *The National Service Framework for Older People*. London: Department of Health.

Department of Health (2002) *Mental Health Policy Implementation Guide: adult inpatient care provision*. London: Department of Health.

Department of Health (2006) *From Values to Actions: the Chief Nursing Officer's review of mental health nursing*. London: Department of Health.

Department of Health (2008) *Attitudes to Mental Illness Research Report*. London: Department of Health.

Department of Health (2009) *Dignity in Care*. London: Department of Health. www.dhcarenetworks.org.uk/dignityincare/index.cfm (accessed 13 October 2010).

Dodds P, Bowles N (2001) Dismantling formal observation and refocusing nursing activity in acute in-patient psychiatry. *Journal of Psychiatric and Mental Health Nursing* 8: 173–88.

European Parliament (2006) *Improving the Mental Health of the Population: a Strategy for the European Union*. www.europarl.europa.eu/oeil/file.jsp?id=5319462 (accessed 13 October 2010).

Mental Health Act Commission (2009) *Coercion and Consent: monitoring the Mental Health Act*. London: Mental Health Act Commission.

Mind (2004) *Ward Watch: Mind's campaign to improve hospital conditions for mental health patients*. London: Mind.

Moylan LB (2009) Physical restraint in acute care psychiatry. *Journal of Psychosocial Nursing and Mental Health Services* 47(3): 41–7.

National Institute for Mental Health in England (2004) *The Ten Essential Shared Capabilities: a framework for the whole of the mental health workforce.* London: National Institute for Mental Health in England.

National Patient Safety Agency (2006) *With Safety in Mind: mental health services and patient safety.* London: National Patient Safety Agency.

Nolan P (1999) *A History of Mental Health Nursing.* Cheltenham: Nelson Thornes Ltd.

Parsons C (2008) The dignity of risk. *Australian Nursing Journal* **15**(9): 28.

Penhale B (2008) Elder abuse in the United Kingdom. *Journal of Elder Abuse and Neglect* **20**(2): 151–68.

Read J, Barker S (1996) *Not Just Sticks and Stones: a survey of the stigma, taboos and discrimination experienced by people with mental health problems.* London: Mind.

Rethink (2006) *Stigma Shout: service user and carer experiences of stigma and discrimination.* London: Rethink.

Sainsbury Centre for Mental Health (1998) *Acute Problems: a survey of the quality of care in acute psychiatric wards.* London: Sainsbury Centre for Mental Health.

Sainsbury Centre for Mental Health (2002) *An Executive Briefing on Adult Acute Inpatient Care for People with Mental Health Problems.* London: Sainsbury Centre for Mental Health.

Sainsbury Centre for Mental Health (2004) *Acute Care: a national survey of adult psychiatric wards in England.* London: Sainsbury Centre for Mental Health.

Sayce L (2000) *From Psychiatric Patient to Citizen: overcoming discrimination and social exclusion.* London: Macmillan Press.

TNS for Shift, CSIP (2007) *Attitudes to Mental Illness in England.* London: TNS.

van der Merwe M, Bowers L, Jones J et al (2009) Locked doors in acute inpatient psychiatry: a literature review. *Journal of Psychiatric and Mental Health Nursing* **16**(3): 293–9.

Woodbridge K, Fullford B (2005) *Whose Values? A workbook for values-based practice in mental health care.* London: Sainsbury Centre for Mental Health.

CHAPTER 14

Dignity and people with learning disabilities

Bob Hallawell

INTRODUCTION

This chapter will explore specific aspects of dignity related to the concept of learning disability and the particular context of the promotion of dignity within services designed to meet the needs of people with learning disabilities.

Learning disability is defined for the purposes of this chapter as a significant impairment of intellectual functioning with significant limitations in adaptive behaviour as expressed in conceptual, social, and practical adaptive skills, which are evident during the developmental period (prior to the age of 18 years) (Department of Health [DH], 2001). Learning disability is not to be confused with learning difficulty, as more broadly defined in education. Other terms that may be used globally to represent learning disability include 'intellectual disability' and 'mental retardation'.

People with learning disabilities have experienced a contravention of their dignity through a number of historical and social manifestations, and such breaches of dignity continue to this day. The origins and nature of such breaches will be explored here, together with contemporary ideas that seek to enable people with learning disabilities to lead dignified and rewarding lives. The discussion will be founded on the notion of dignity as an individual feeling of worthiness and respect (NHS Modernisation Agency, 2003) or, as the Royal College of Nursing stated:

> Dignity is concerned with how people feel, think and behave in relation to the worth or value of themselves and others. To treat someone with dignity is to treat them as being of worth, in a way that is respectful of them as valued individuals (RCN, 2008, p.6, reproduced with permission from the Royal College of Nursing).

LEARNING OUTCOMES

After reading this chapter you will be able to:

➤ explain how historical and social influences created devalued identities for people with learning disabilities, and a consequent lack of dignity in their lives

➤ appreciate how social policy may both hinder and promote dignity in the lives of people with learning disabilities

➤ identify contemporary thinking about the promotion of dignity within health and social care settings for people with learning disabilities

➤ identify how individuals and services may promote dignity through their thinking and actions.

SOCIAL INFLUENCES AND SOCIETAL IMPRESSIONS

Social policy for people with learning disabilities in the latter part of the 19th century and the early decades of the 20th century was partly driven by segregationist principles that underpinned the eugenics movement of the time. These segregationist principles were themselves based on three beliefs: first, that intelligence and ability were inherited; secondly, that people with a learning disability bred at a faster rate than the rest of society; and thirdly, that there were strong links between 'feeble-mindedness' and major social problems (Emerson, 2005). 'It was as a social grouping and as a social problem that individuals with a learning disability were perceived, treated and ultimately constructed' (McClimens, 2005, p.43). Within such a socially constructed identity, people with learning disabilities were not afforded rights to choice, decision making or involvement in the nature of service delivery. Thus, social policy based on eugenic principles served to stigmatise specific groups of individuals and denied them their basic human rights (Richardson, 2005).

Now carry out Reflective activity 14.1.

Reflective activity 14.1

➤ How important is inclusion, choice and the right to make decisions to you?

➤ In the absence of such factors, is it possible to feel worthy and respected?

Economic imperatives also drove the legislation for, classification of and segregation of madness (and other deviance) in the 19th century. Classifications of disability can be linked back to the 'deserving' and 'undeserving' poor criteria established in the Poor Law Reforms of 1834. Thus, industrialisation and a dominant capitalist ideology resulted in the social exclusion of people with physical or mental impairments in the 18th and 19th centuries (Richardson, 2005). A political response to this exclusion and marginalisation was to institutionalise provision for the disabled, first in workhouses and later in specialised institutions. Within these closed, segregated and often authoritarian environments, disabled people 'were socialised into a view of themselves as sick, helpless, inferior and in need of help and care to survive' (Goble, 2004, p.41).

Chapter 2's exploration of dignity introduced 'place, people and process' as factors affecting dignity. Table 14.1 presents how the socialisation process engendered by institutionalisation was characterised by a lack of dignity expressed in place, people and process. After reading the table carry out Reflective activity 14.2.

Table 14.1 Institutions and a lack of dignity (RCN, 2010)

Place	People	Process
• Little or no privacy in the environment	• The promotion of personal identity was largely absent, e.g. shared clothing, shared toiletries, shared living space	• Rigid, prescribed regimes, e.g. drinks at set times; fixed bedtimes; fixed bathing times
• Barren, impoverished environments	• People had very little in terms of personal possessions	• Lack of choice
• Institutions/hospitals were often situated at a distance from the person's home, family and friends	• The language of the institution was often stigmatising and undignified, staff to patient and patient to patient	• Families had to apply in writing to obtain permission to take their relative out of the grounds of the institution
• Restricted or no access to the outside world		
• All resources, activities, experiences were supplied within the institution by the institution		

Reflective activity 14.2

➤ Do the characteristics of the institution (*see* Table 14.1) sound familiar to you today?

➤ Can you think of other examples from your own experiences of large institutions within society, for example, schools or hospitals?

A lack of dignity within institutional settings has also been reflected in the personal accounts of those who lived within the institutions. For example, Atkinson and Williams's (1990) book of narratives from people with learning disabilities has provided vivid examples. Peter Stevens (p.191) related the constraints and authoritarianism of hospital life: 'You have to be told what to do in hospital'; 'You rely on the food being dished up and I don't like it'. When he was young, he said: 'we always had to go to bed early' and he further said of the charge nurses and nurses: 'I have the strange feeling that they think they are the ones that know better.' Ronnie Gaukrodger (p.198) explained how they were not allowed to talk at the table and that on one occasion, while sitting with others around the table, he started talking, with the result that a nurse: 'just came and pulled me in the pantry, and walloped me on the back of me earhole'. He went on to say that she 'threw a basin at me and split me head open'. The nurse then told him: 'you don't say anything to the doctor'. Ronnie described feeling 'very frightened. I couldn't say anything'.

Now carry out Reflective activity 14.3.

Reflective activity 14.3

➤ Is it likely that such provision and the resultant self-perception will promote worthiness and respect?

➤ How much do social environments determine your feelings of dignity and respect? Can you identify any experiences that were either positive or negative in nature?

IDENTITY, NORMALISATION AND PERSONALISATION

People with learning disabilities who experienced the effects of institutional living have, through such accounts, enabled us to better understand both their personal and social identities. Personal identity may be formed through experience – a sense of belonging, of being loved and valued; being treated as an adult; and being able to value one's self (Atkinson and Williams, 1990). Such characteristics sit well with the idea of dignity as individual feelings of worthiness and respect. However, personal identity is not developed without interaction with a social world that further enables the establishment of a social identity. Social identity may be defined as:

> . . . the ways in which collectivities and individuals are distinguished in their relations with other collectivities or individuals; the establishment, signification and organisation of relationships of similarity and difference between collectivities and individuals . . . (Jenkins, 1998, p.6, reproduced with permission from Cambridge University Press).

The manner in which identities, roles and labels are negotiated and constructed will determine who is considered disabled (Goodley, 2004). Historically, people with learning disabilities have been represented within society under a number of identities. These include the subhuman, the holy innocent, the sick, the eternal child, the vagabond, the ineducable, the defective, the idiot, the mentally subnormal and the mentally handicapped (Gates, 1997; Grant *et al*, 2005).

Both personal and social identities develop as a result of the socialisation processes experienced by the individual, and individuals may inherit included or excluded identities (Borland and Ramcharan, 1997). The adoption of certain social roles, the achievement of a valued status and the acquisition of useful skills or accomplishments all contribute to the individual's social identity (Atkinson and Williams, 1990). People with learning disabilities may at times have struggled to establish valued personal and social identities in the face of stigmatisation by both society and powerful and articulate individuals. Powerful individuals may set the tone for dialogue about less powerful individuals. For example, identities such as 'able-bodied' and 'normal' are constructed by those who wield power as a result of status and authority conferred by legitimated knowledge (Thomas, 2004). However, Ward (2000), referring to earlier work by Lukes (1974), argued that one should refrain from solely focusing on the behaviour of specific decision makers but also consider how systems may both define and work against people's interests. This form of power '. . . is not only the capacity to impose (if necessary in the face of opposition) but [. . .] also the capacity to set the terms of debate' (Ward, 2000, p.50).

Calhoun (1994) argued that where such dominant discourses repress, delegitimate or devalue a particular identity, a fundamental response may be to claim value for those labelled by a given category (for example, learning disabilities). Inclusion in society is central to the development of self-concept and identity, and if subject to exclusionary experiences then: 'it is likely that the person will be socialised into an excluded self-concept and identity' (Borland and Ramcharan, 1997, p.88). Gates (1997) further notes how social incompetence may result from the segregation and devalued lifestyles to be found within the learning disability hospitals that provided care during the 20th century. People with learning disabilities may continue to be seen as people who have to be cared for, and thus they are disregarded and excluded and seen as 'the other' (Walmsley, 2000). Mackenzie (2005) argues that 'learning disabilities has come to be understood as a socially constructed condition to which the most helpful response is social inclusion' (p.47). Thus, inclusive identities, with other groups and individuals, are dependent upon inclusionary socialisation processes.

Now carry out Reflective activity 14.4.

Reflective activity 14.4

➤ Can you think of situations through which your involvement gave you a sense of being included?
➤ What strategies did you adopt in order to become included?
➤ How dependent were you on others to include you?
➤ Did you alter any aspects of your personal identity in order to take on a new social identity?

The advent of normalisation philosophy, participatory research and the self-advocacy movement in the late 20th century and the early 21st century were crucial in enabling people with learning disabilities to be heard and to enable them to adopt valued social roles (Atkinson, 2005). Normalisation theory originally developed partly as a reaction to institutional care and proposed that people with learning disabilities should be enabled to live ordinary lives, such as those experienced by other members of society. The theory was based on three central tenets: first, that people with learning disabilities should experience the normal rhythms of life such as those based on work, play and a varied day; secondly, that there should be a separation of life functions, in contrast to institutional life where often all functions would be carried out in one ward; and thirdly, that service provision should be based on culturally valued analogues, that is, services should be based on culturally valued ways of meeting the needs of people who use services (Cocks, 2001). Later conceptualisations of normalisation (Wolfensberger and Thomas, 1983) acknowledged social identity in emphasising how people with learning disabilities were portrayed and perceived by the public. These conceptualisations articulated the need to develop valued social roles for this group of people (Means and Smith, 1998, p.72), while Williams and Tyne (1988) noted the need to develop 'value based services' in order to militate against negative social values and the concomitant negative life experiences of people with disabilities.

The 1960s also saw an extension of the notion of rights to more 'marginal' groups within society, including people with disabilities (Emerson, 2005). Professional ideologies were also influenced in the 1960s and 1970s by the United Nations's (1948) declarations on human rights and the rights of mentally retarded persons (Office of the United Nations High Commissioner for Human Rights, 1971). These developments built upon the influence of parental pressure groups, the disability rights movement, and social research during the middle decades of the 20th century. Such developments had led to the awareness that people with learning disabilities may grow and develop with the removal of adverse social circumstances, such as institutionalisation and social exclusion (Richardson, 2005). Walker (1997) argued that services delivered within a user-centred framework would '. . . be organised to respect the users' right to self-determination, normalisation and dignity . . .' (p.216). Dawson (1997) also noted that active participation in services was occurring because people with learning disabilities were seen to be of equal worth to non-learning disabled people and were valued as expert consultants because of their direct experience of services. Thus, the personal and social identities of people with learning disabilities had undergone a transformation leading to a new sense of worth and value and a new sense of dignity based upon respect for the individual and their unique expertise.

DIGNITY, HEALTH AND SOCIAL CARE

The physical environment, service cultures, the attitudes and behaviours of the care team, and the manner in which care is delivered may individually or together determine whether dignity is diminished or promoted (RCN, 2010). The notion of dignity applies equally to those who may lack intellectual capacity as it does to individuals who are held to be mentally competent. This requires that care staff treat people of any health status in any setting with dignity. Now carry out Reflective activity 14.5.

Reflective activity 14.5

➤ Think about your previous experiences of healthcare.
➤ What aspects of that care led you feel that you were treated with dignity?

People with learning disabilities (RCN, 2010) identified the following characteristics:
➤ an understanding of their health needs
➤ being treated with respect.
➤ people taking the time to get to know them
➤ having choices and making decisions
➤ feeling safe.

The presence or absence of dignified care may lead to a range of feelings and outcomes for people. The earlier discussions in this chapter noted how people with learning disabilities felt devalued, controlled and excluded by the conditions under which care was provided at the time. The provision of the right social circumstances, environments and approaches to care, and the resultant promotion of dignity can lead to alternative outcomes and feelings (*see* Table 14.2).

Table 14.2 Outcomes and feelings associated with the presence or absence of dignity (RCN, 2010)

Dignity present	Dignity absent
In control	Lack of control
Valued	Devalued
Confident	Lacking confidence
Comfortable	Uncomfortable
Able to make decisions	Unable to make decisions
	Humiliation
	Embarrassment
	Shame

Although it is important to treat all individuals with dignity, there are some particular measures or strategies that may need to be put into place to promote the dignity of people with learning disabilities. There are some particularly damning reports of the experiences of people with learning disabilities when they access mainstream healthcare facilities (Disability Rights Commission, 2006; Mencap, 2007; Michael, 2008). The commonly reported difficulties include:

➤ discrimination against individuals
➤ healthcare professionals who do not understand the law about capacity and consent to treatment
➤ healthcare professionals do not always see the lives of people with a learning disability as worth saving
➤ assumptions made about individuals by professionals, with no assessment to substantiate them
➤ lack of communication between professionals, the individual and their carers
➤ difficulty for people with learning disabilities in accessing services
➤ staff who lack knowledge and skills in working with people with learning disabilities
➤ abuse of individuals and neglect by services, sometimes leading to unnecessary deaths (Mencap, 2007; RCN, 2010).

People with learning disabilities may also find healthcare particularly difficult for a number of reasons. It is likely that they will find it difficult to explain what they are experiencing in terms of pain or discomfort, and they may also struggle to make a rapid adjustment to changing routines and environments that may be part of healthcare services. Healthcare staff may not fully understand their cognitive, health and personal needs and the individuals may have themselves experienced poor healthcare in the past (Hebron, 2009).

Read through Michael's scenario in Reflective activity 14.6 and then consider the questions that follow.

Reflective activity 14.6 Scenario – Michael goes to the hospital

Michael is a 22-year-old man with Down's syndrome, who lives at home with his family. He has moderate learning disabilities and is capable of managing some of his daily life independently, for example eating and personal hygiene. He has some speech but others often find it difficult to understand what he is saying. Staff at the day resource that he attends have been working with him to help him use a sign language known as Makaton. It is known that Michael likes to organise his life around specific routines and activities and he has particular possessions that he likes to keep around him at all times.

Michael has been admitted to hospital by his consultant for cardiac surgery.

➤ What information would be needed to support Michael's care? Where might such information come from?
➤ How would you establish what Michael's support needs are?
➤ How might you communicate with Michael?
➤ How might you give information to Michael about the routines and practices within the hospital?
➤ Might Michael's need to have his possessions with him pose any problems? Would there be any strategies that might help with this situation?

Resource
You may find the following resource helpful in answering the questions: *Working Together: easy steps to improving how people with a learning disability are supported when in hospital:* www.library.nhs.uk/learningdisabilities/ViewResource.aspx?resID=305541

Michael's situation might raise some questions that are difficult to answer, but there are some very practical steps suggested by both people with learning disabilities and learning disabilities professionals that may be taken in order to provide dignified care to Michael and other people with learning disabilities. For example:

➤ all nurses and support staff should have training about people with learning disabilities

➤ healthcare staff should be familiar with any policies and procedures for the safeguarding of vulnerable adults and children

➤ people with learning disabilities should have regular health checks and each have a health action plan that can be used as information for others. They might also have something called a health passport or health profile that provides information on health needs, choices, likes and dislikes, reactions to medication or pain and required levels of support

➤ community teams for people with learning disabilities should give other nurses information and support

➤ it should be established whether there is a learning disability liaison nurse or health facilitator for the hospital

➤ nurses should understand their responsibilities with respect to capacity and consent. They should thus appreciate the key principles of the Mental Capacity Act

➤ people with learning disabilities should be given information and help about how to stay well, such as eating healthily or exercising. This information should be provided in understandable formats as required, for example, pictures and symbols

➤ the person with the learning disability, and not only the carers or other staff, should be spoken to about their needs. They should be addressed in the manner preferred by the person

➤ people with learning disabilities should be included at all stages of the care planning process. They may need to know what to expect, what might happen and how they may feel

➤ people with learning disabilities may require more intensive preparation. A preadmission visit might therefore be arranged to identify potential risks, to establish levels of dependency and to define the necessary levels of support. Balancing the need to manage risks against the person's independence is crucial to providing a safe and dignified experience

➤ nurses should seek to establish what the person can do for themselves – not assume a lack of capability. They should also be asked what support they do need and in what form that support might be best provided

➤ more time should be allowed for consultations/assessments – double appointments may be necessary. Also, more time should be allowed for self-care

➤ private, accessible and clean environments should be provided, with understandable signs and/or information.

➤ communication should use simple, everyday language and concrete terms rather than abstract ideas. Consider the use of photographs, pictures and symbols to assist communication

➤ new events or procedures and the reason for the change should be explained. This may require pictorial or symbolic forms of communication in addition to verbal language
➤ information about the staff and their roles should be provided
➤ if giving medication, people with learning disabilities should be told:
  – what it is for
  – why it should be taken
  – how it will help
  – about the side-effects
  – the information in a format that is easy to understand
  – how to take the medication
➤ feedback should be provided to the person on procedures and progress and their particular response to the treatment
➤ particular discharge arrangements that may need to be made to support the person in their home should be thought about
➤ a learning disabilities champion should be established within the service area, who can be a source of information and advice to the staff team (Hebron, 2009; RCN, 2010).

Dignified care for people with learning disabilities need not be an extremely complex episode if some of these practical steps are taken before, during and after access to healthcare services and professionals.

CONCLUSION

People with learning disabilities may experience a lack of dignity fostered by historical and social impressions of their worth and value to society. A devalued personal and social identity may in turn lead to dehumanising practices and service provision that may result in undignified lifestyles and, in the worst instances, abuse, neglect and unnecessary deaths. Changes in thinking, policy and practice have led to the emergence of new, valued social roles for people with learning disabilities that foster choice, respect, rights and dignity. An awareness of this, aligned with some specific policy imperatives and new models of care within health and social systems, may lead to the enhancement of dignified practice by health and social care professionals. This, in turn, may result in people with learning disabilities having a new-found sense of personal worth. People with learning disabilities are not a homogenous group, and, as such, dignity can be promoted through the recognition of each person as an individual with a unique personality, history and range of abilities (RCN, 2010).

REFERENCES

Atkinson D (2005) Narratives and people with learning disabilities. In: Grant G, Goward P, Richardson M, Ramcharan P (eds) *Learning Disability – A Life Cycle Approach to Valuing People.* Maidenhead: Open University Press, pp.7–27.

Atkinson D, Williams F (eds) (1990) *Know Me As I Am: an anthology of prose, poetry and art by people with learning difficulties.* London: Hodder and Stoughton.

Borland J, Ramcharan P (1997) Empowerment in informal settings – the themes. In: Ramcharan P, Roberts G, Grant G, Borland J (eds) *Empowerment in Everyday Life – Learning Disability.* London: Jessica Kingsley Publishers, pp.88–97.

Calhoun C (ed) (1994) *Social Theory and the Politics of Identity.* Oxford: Blackwell.

Cocks E (2001) Normalisation and social role valorisation: guidance for human service development. *Hong Kong Journal of Psychiatry* **11**(1): 12–16.

Dawson P (1997) Service planning and people with learning disabilities. *British Journal of Nursing* **6**(2): 70.

Department of Health (2001) *Valuing People: a new strategy for learning disability for the 21st century.* London: The Stationery Office.

Disability Rights Commission (2006) *Equal Treatment: closing the gap – a formal investigation into physical health inequalities experienced by people with learning disabilities and/or mental health problems.* London: Disability Rights Commission.

Emerson E (2005) Models of service delivery. In: Grant G, Goward P, Richardson M, Ramcharan P (eds) *Learning Disability – A Life Cycle Approach to Valuing People.* Maidenhead: Open University Press, pp.108–27.

Gates B (1997) The nature of learning disability. In: Gates B, Beacock C (eds) *Dimensions of Learning Disability.* London: Baillière Tindall, pp.3–25.

Goble C (2004) Dependency, independence and normality. In: Swain J, French S, Barnes C, Thomas C (eds) *Disabling Barriers – Enabling Environments.* London: Sage Publications, pp.41–6.

Goodley D (2004) Who is disabled? Exploring the scope of the social model of disability. In: Swain J, French S, Barnes C, Thomas C (eds) *Disabling Barriers – Enabling Environment.* London: Sage Publications, pp.118–24.

Grant G, Goward P, Richardson M, Ramcharan, P (eds) (2005) *Learning Disability – A life Cycle Approach to Valuing People.* Maidenhead: Open University Press.

Hebron C (2009) Working together to ensure equal healthcare for all. *Learning Disability Practice* **12**(6): 27–30.

Jenkins R (ed) (1998) *Questions of Competence – Culture, Classification and Intellectual Disability.* Cambridge: University Press.

Lukes S (1974) *Power: a radical view.* London: Macmillan.

MacKenzie F (2005) The roots of biomedical diagnosis. In: Grant G, Goward P, Richardson M, Ramcharan P (eds) *Learning Disability – A Life Cycle Approach to Valuing People.* Maidenhead: Open University Press, pp.47–65.

McClimens A (2005) From vagabonds to Victorian values. In: Grant G, Goward P, Richardson M, Ramcharan P (eds) *Learning Disability – A Life Cycle Approach to Valuing People.* Maidenhead: Open University Press, pp.28–46.

Means R, Smith R (1998) *Community Care – Policy and Practice.* Basingstoke: Macmillan Press Ltd.

Mencap (2007) *Death by Indifference: following up the Treat me Right! Report.* London: Mencap.

Michael J (2008) *Healthcare For All: report of the independent inquiry into access to healthcare for people with learning disabilities.* London: Aldridge Press.

NHS Modernisation Agency (2003) *The Essence of Care – patient focused benchmarks for clinical governance.* London: NHS Modernisation Agency. www.dh.gov.uk/dr_consum_dh/groups/dh_digitalassets/@dh/@en/documents/digitalasset/dh_4127915.pdf (accessed 13 October 2010).

Office of the United Nations High Commissioner for Human Rights (1971) *Declaration on the Rights of Mentally Retarded Persons.* www2.ohchr.org/english/law/res2856.htm (accessed 13 October 2010).

Richardson M (2005) Critiques of segregation and eugenics. In: Grant G, Goward P, Richardson M, Ramcharan P (eds) *Learning Disability – A Life Cycle Approach to Valuing People.* Maidenhead: Open University Press, pp.66–89.

Royal College of Nursing (2008) *Dignity: at the heart of everything we do.* London: Royal College of Nursing. www.rcn.org.uk/newsevents/campaigns/dignity (accessed 17 August 2010).

Royal College of Nursing (2010) *Dignity in Healthcare for People with Learning Disabilities – RCN guidance.* London: Royal College of Nursing.

Thomas C (2004) Disability and impairment. In: Swain J, French S, Barnes C, Thomas C (eds) *Disabling Barriers – Enabling Environments.* London: Sage Publications, pp.21–7.

United Nations (1948) *The Universal Declaration of Human Rights.* www.un.org/en/documents/udhr/ (accessed 13 October 2010).

Walker A (1997) Community care policy: from consensus to conflict. In: Bornat J, Johnson J, Pereira C, Pilgrim D, Williams F (eds) *Community Care: a reader.* London: Macmillan Press Ltd, pp.196–220.

Walmsley J (2000) Caring: a place in the world?' In: Johnson K, Traustadottir R (eds) *Women with Intellectual Disabilities: finding a place in the world.* London: Jessica Kingsley, pp.191–212.

Ward D (2000) Totem not token – groupwork as a vehicle for user participation. In: Kemshall H, Littlechild R (eds) *User Involvement and Participation in Social Care.* London: Jessica Kingsley, pp.45–64.

Williams P, Tyne A (1998) Exploring values as the basis for service development. In: Towell D (ed) *An Ordinary Life in Practice: developing comprehensive community-based services for people with learning difficulties.* London: King's Fund Publishing, pp.23–31.

Wolfensberger W, Thomas S (1983) *PASSING: Program Analysis of Service Systems Implementing Normalisation Goals.* Toronto: National Institute on Mental Retardation.

SECTION 3
Developing dignity in healthcare

CHAPTER 15

Education to promote dignity in healthcare

Liz Cotrel-Gibbons and Milika Ruth Matiti

INTRODUCTION

The public's desire for healthcare that promotes the dignity of clients has become an overt demand – it is therefore vital that healthcare professionals are formally educated about what dignity means and how it can be promoted. This chapter will focus on the approaches to education that can be employed to promote dignity in care and is aimed at both students and educators in health-care. There is specific reference to pre-registration nurse education but the content is also applicable to other students receiving their initial education in healthcare.

In the first section of the chapter the rationale for 'values education' in nurs-ing and healthcare and the position of dignity within 'values education' will be presented. Challenges to dignity education will be identified. The educational theories of deep learning, andragogy, constructivism and transformative learn-ing, and their relevance for dignity education, are discussed. This will provide a solid theoretical foundation for the section on the implementation of educa-tional strategies.

The second section uses the six questions posed by Kipling in 1902 (1989) as a framework: What? Why? When? How? Where? Who? An example of a programme for dignity education is outlined and specific examples of how to implement this programme are given. Some of the content is based on our per-sonal experiences. Reflective exercises are included to enable readers to experi-ence and evaluate some of the strategies.

LEARNING OUTCOMES

By the end of the chapter you will be able to:
➤ identify the rationale for 'values education'
➤ be aware of the challenges to 'values education'
➤ discuss the relevance of deep learning, andragogy, constructivism and transformative learning to dignity education

➤ discuss the implementation of values/dignity education
➤ experience and evaluate learning exercises.

A CASE FOR DIGNITY IN THE CURRICULUM

As stated in previous chapters of this book, dignity is a value; it is more than an attitude, knowledge or a skill. A value is a belief that guides behaviour and provides criteria for making choices (Vezeau, 2006). Dignity does not stand alone – other relevant values in healthcare include integrity, empathy, compassion, caring and respect. However, dignity has been claimed to be a core value of nursing practice. In Norway, Fagermoen (1997) investigated values embedded in nursing practice by asking 767 qualified nurses: 'What is most meaningful in your work as a nurse?'. The findings indicated that dignity was a core value for nurses when caring for patients. Fagermoen (1997) found that the other values the nurses identified, such as integrity, either arose from the value of dignity or were aimed at preserving dignity, for example privacy.

The values of integrity (Teeri *et al*, 2008), empathy (Fahrenwald *et al*, 2005; Manthey, 2008), compassion (Fahrenwald *et al*, 2005; Kalb and O'Connor-Von, 2007; Cornwell and Goodrich, 2009), caring (Fahrenwald *et al*, 2005) and respect (Kalb and O'Connor-Von, 2007; Manthey, 2008; Teeri *et al*, 2008; Cornwell and Goodrich, 2009) are all bound together; if one is missing from healthcare practice, the ability to promote dignity is compromised. It therefore follows that these values need to be incorporated in the curriculum.

Raya (1990) argues that universities have a responsibility to teach values, not just knowledge, because values direct the use of knowledge and encourage respect for truth and for the worth and rights of other people. Hoover's study (2002) demonstrated that values education enhanced students' knowledge and intent to practise in a caring way. Improvement in the care experiences of patients and their families is the main aim of values education. The ways in which values are incorporated in the education of healthcare professionals indicate how the promotion of dignity may be learned.

The need for explicit dignity education for nurses is recommended by many authors including Johnston *et al* (2004) in Australia, Jacelon *et al* (2004) in the United States of America, and Matiti (2002), Tschudin (2004) and Woogara (2005) in the United Kingdom (UK). The necessity for dignity to be explicit in educational programmes is supported by the American Association of Colleges of Nursing (1998), which identified five core professional nursing values – altruism, autonomy, human dignity, integrity and social justice. In the UK, the Nursing and Midwifery Council (NMC; 2007) published the 'Essential Skills Clusters', with one section on 'care, compassion and communication', which specifically encompasses dignity.

However, there are some challenges to values education that need to be kept in mind by healthcare educators. The first challenge is that dignity is, as has been discussed in earlier chapters, difficult to define and subjective. As a consequence, lecturers might have different perceptions of dignity, which can pose problems when considering how to incorporate dignity into educational programmes. A second challenge is the current lack of literature and evidence on the implementation of values education in pre-registration curricula. A third is the limited amount of time available due to a packed curriculum (Warburton, 2003). Vezeau (2006) identifies that values education is difficult as it raises potentially uncomfortable questions and may challenge self-image. Despite all these challenges, it is our contention that healthcare education should aim to develop knowledge, skills and appropriate attitudes among students in relation to the concept of dignity. The next section identifies and discusses the educational theories that can be utilised when teaching about dignity.

EDUCATIONAL APPROACHES AND THEORIES

When reviewing the literature on how the concept of dignity is transmitted to others, there are three main approaches:

➤ *ethical*: moral judgements on how people ought to be treated
➤ *political*: legal rights as in the Human Rights Act (1998)
➤ *spiritual*: as a dimension of the person's self-concept.

While all three are underpinned by values and have merit, the majority of nursing literature focuses on the ethical approach. This chapter draws on all three approaches but focuses on application to practice.

There are a number of educational theories but four will be outlined and their relevance to dignity education discussed: deep learning, andragogy, constructivism and transformative learning.

Deep learning

Dignity is both a multifaceted and a personal concept. Each person has a personal concept of dignity which shapes their attitudes and actions. Healthcare professionals interact with clients and, in addition to enacting their own concept of dignified behaviour, have to develop an understanding of each client's dignity and then provide conditions to promote the dignity of that client. In order to achieve this level of practice, healthcare professionals must develop an understanding of what dignity means both to themselves and to others, such as clients. This can lead to a dilemma, as values are embedded in a person's self-concept and are difficult to change. Any challenge to a person's values causes a need for them to review core aspects of themselves, which may lead to dissonance between who they are and who they feel/think they should be. A specific example is the debate about what constitutes a dignified death. On the one hand, there is the argument for the sanctity of life and promotion of dignity through palliative care, while on the other there is the right to self-determination including choosing when and how to die.

In educational terms, developing this understanding requires deep as opposed to surface learning (Clare, 2007). Beattie *et al* (1997) define deep learning as 'learning with understanding'. The distinction between deep and surface learning was first made in 1976 by Marton and Saljo. Surface learning is identified as being extrinsically motivated, passive and requiring reproduction of knowledge, while deep learning is an 'intrinsically motivated process of personalised meaning construction'. Clare (2007) used deep learning strategies with her social work students by encouraging them to use a reflective journal and facilitating dialogue between the student and the content, other students and the teacher. She found that her students developed critical thinking about practice and themselves as practitioners, which she attributed to employing deep learning strategies. The students felt that they had 'a stronger foundation for entering the professional practice arena' (p.443).

It is, however, acknowledged that learning about dignity may also have extrinsic motivators such as health and social policy and practice guides, for example Dignity in Care (Department of Health, 2006). These motivators need to be examined, analysed and critiqued before being included in the students' personalised meaning constructions. Merely presenting policies leads to surface learning, what Beattie *et al* (1997) would identify as rote learning, with limited ability to instigate professional practice.

According to Entwistle (2000), the intention of deep learning is to extract meaning; this requires the student to be actively involved in their learning. Pask (1988) identified two strands to deep learning: first the holist strategy, which involves looking for patterns and principles; and secondly the serialist strategy, which uses evidence and logic. Both of these strategies are relevant when enabling students to develop an understanding and application of a complex and difficult-to-define concept such as dignity. The holist strategy encourages reflection on students' personal concepts and practice experiences; the serialist strategy uses research and planning processes to support students in making changes to their own practice.

Key concepts that are relevant to deep learning are:
- internal motivation of the student
- active learning – engagement with the topic (Warburton, 2003)
- provision of opportunities to develop enhanced personal meaning (Entwistle, 2000; Warburton, 2003)
- relevance of teaching – from the student's perspective (Warburton, 2003).
- self-assessment to guide the learning process (Sandberg and Barnard, 1997).

These concepts can be applied to dignity education in the following ways. Internal motivation can be stimulated by encouraging students to analyse their own personal concept of dignity and to consider what makes them feel respected. In the authors' experiences, the student's inbuilt desire to care for others is a strong motivator for promoting dignity for patients. The learning activities that are incorporated into an educational programme need to enable students to critically analyse and reflect on their personal attitudes, knowledge and skills, as well as on the literature and policies. This provides students with the opportunity to develop their personal concept of dignity and their role in promoting dignity for patients. Focusing on their role ensures that the learning has professional relevance for students. In addition, the opportunity to develop an aspect of practice through action planning, and then evaluate the effectiveness of how this has led to service improvement, incorporates all five of the key concepts.

Andragogy

In the education of healthcare professionals, the philosophy of andragogy needs to run alongside the principle of deep learning. The students are adults, and therefore an andragogical approach needs to underpin all teaching strategies; this is a fundamental way of treating students with respect and so maintaining their dignity. In turn, being valued themselves will reinforce the importance of promoting the dignity of others. The elements of andragogy that are particularly relevant for values education are:

➤ the adult's accumulation of life experiences, which can act as a resource for learning, for example, their personal experience of dignity or of dignity promotion in practice

➤ the adult's readiness to learn is related to what they need to know or do in their life; for example, how will learning about dignity help to develop their practice? (Jarvis, 1987; Quinn and Hughes, 2007).

In addition, Quinn and Hughes (2007) and Henschke and Cooper (2009) suggest that an adult is predominantly internally motivated, for example, by job satisfaction, as opposed to relying on approval from others. However, this may not always be the case in professional education when learning is assessed by the same people who are facilitating the adult's learning; gaining these facilitators' formal approval becomes paramount in order to pass the course (Entwistle, 2000; Warburton, 2003). An example that relates to dignity is the healthcare student placing a higher priority on working quickly rather than on respecting the patient's need for compassionate communication. The role of assessment in values education therefore needs to be considered carefully if it is to promote and not restrict learning.

Two further learning theories that have relevance to values education are:
➤ constructivist learning
➤ transformative learning.

Both of these theories are from the cognitive school of learning and focus on internal mental processes, not just demonstrated behaviours (Mezirow, 2000).

Constructivism

Constructivist learning is based on the work of Piaget who rejected the idea of the teacher pouring knowledge into the empty student vessel (Weinberg and Weinberg, 1983). Constructivism assumes that learners build their knowledge by identifying meanings from their own experiences. This requires active learners with the ability to use past and present experiences, thus linking to both deep learning and andragogy. In relation to dignity education, constructive learning can be facilitated by asking the students trigger questions about their own experiences or actions and then asking the students to consider how this affects their professional practice.

Transformative learning

Transformative learning is based on Mezirow's work (Williams, 2001). This takes account of the ideas of constructivism, moving on to use the meanings that the learner identifies to transform their view of others or self and to guide future action. This is vital in practice-based professions. Strategies to promote transformative learning may set out to challenge existing 'frames of reference', as in Rush's (2008) study. Rush examined the impact of employing mental health service users to teach nursing on the nursing students' attitudes about the potential capabilities of these mental health service users. The students' previous experiences of mental health service users had been as providers of their care rather than as recipients of their knowledge. In relation to promoting dignity, working with clients to formulate a dignity charter would enable students to work in partnership with clients. This challenges the usual relationship of caregiver and recipient and enables students to work in new ways. Providing opportunities for students to experience the world from the clients' perspectives, reflecting on how that makes them feel and then identifying actions that they could undertake to promote dignity, would also be transformative.

In order to evaluate the teaching strategies, Reflective activity 15.1 will help you to understand the relevance of these educational theories.

An example would be:

> My experience relates to riding a horse. I am not a confident rider. I don't believe that I can influence the horse if he doesn't want to listen. I would increase my enjoyment in riding if I felt that I could have more control through working with the

> **Reflective activity 15.1** Educational theories
>
> ➤ Describe an occasion when you felt that you had a good learning experience. It may have been during your professional education, at school/college or be related to a hobby.
> ➤ What was it that made it a good experience? It may have been because you enjoyed the learning activity, or because you learned something or because you felt supported by the teacher or fellow learners.
> ➤ Did this experience use any of the four educational theories discussed in this chapter?

horse. I discussed this with my instructor who knew that I was ready to learn and motivated to improve my riding [key concepts of *deep learning* and *andragogy*]. My instructor knew that I had knowledge of anatomy and movement. She built on this knowledge and related this to my riding technique and the movement of the horse, thereby using my previous life experiences [key concepts of *deep learning*, *andragogy* and *constructivism*]. I was given practical exercises to undertake, so engaged in active learning – both cognitive and psychomotor. Undertaking these exercises enabled me to assess my own progress [key concept of *deep learning*] and to discuss this with my instructor. I was able to identify new meanings from my discussion and experiences, which then led to a transformed view of myself in relation to the meaning of control and risk. This in turn influenced my willingness to extend my riding skills [*transformative learning*].

The theories of andragogy, constructivism and transformative learning all support deep learning, which is crucial if students are to develop their abilities to promote dignity. Sandberg and Barnard (1997) acknowledge that deep learning is difficult and that students require teachers to create learning environments that enable them to actively construct knowledge. Entwistle (2000) suggests that teachers who are student focused and learning orientated, as opposed to teacher focused and content orientated, place a greater emphasis on encouraging students to develop deep levels of understanding. It is with this in mind that the implementation of educational strategies will be discussed in relation to dignity.

IMPLEMENTATION OF EDUCATIONAL STRATEGIES TO PROMOTE DIGNITY IN CARE

In this section the five Ws and one H of Rudyard Kipling (1989) will be used to guide the discussion.

➤ What?
➤ Why?
➤ When?
➤ How?
➤ Where?
➤ Who?

This is a simple framework that ensures that the elements of curriculum planning are considered: content (*what*), rationale for content and method (*why*), logical sequencing (*when*), learning and teaching methods (*how*), learning environment (*where*) and appropriate expertise and skills of the facilitator (*who*). The *why* will be included with each of the other questions in turn.

What needs to be learned?

Education for dignity needs to be included in a wider programme of values education (see Box 15.1 for suggested topics), which includes:
➤ ethics
➤ spirituality
➤ professionalism
➤ attitude formation
➤ communication skills
➤ law and policy relevant to dignity and human rights.

Dignity needs to be considered from three perspectives: personal dignity, patient dignity and the dignity of professional colleagues.

It is acknowledged that the time that can be allocated to specific education about dignity will be limited and that dignity also needs to be incorporated in all sessions that involve interaction with others. However, relying on incorporation alone can lead to the devaluing of dignity as a topic with it being hidden amongst other content – perpetuating the issue of 'dignity being a taken for granted concept'. Therefore specific content that needs to be learned about dignity should be identified.

There needs to be an increase in the complexity of this content to enable the student to develop their cognition and application to practice in relation to dignity. Initially students need to consider their own concept of dignity, explore how it relates to other people's concepts and then move on to reflecting on their own actions. The next stage is to apply their skills and knowledge through working with service users who have a variety of needs and then identifying individual needs within the competing demands of practice. Finally students should develop an understanding of how they can influence colleagues and the organisational culture.

BOX 15.1 *Suggested topics for inclusion in a values education programme*

➤ Altruism – beneficence, non-maleficence
➤ Attitude formation
➤ Autonomy – self-care – choice
➤ Change process
➤ Compassion
➤ Confidentiality
➤ Communication
➤ Consent
➤ Culture – diversity
➤ Dignity
➤ Disability
➤ Discrimination, harassment and exploitation
➤ Diversity
➤ Embarrassment, humiliation, shame
➤ Equality
➤ Ethics – value, worth, personhood
➤ Gender
➤ Mental capacity
➤ Professional code – integrity/accountability
➤ Role modelling
➤ Safeguarding and/or public protection
➤ Sexuality
➤ Social justice
➤ Spirituality
➤ Stigma

Considering the when

In the UK, most pre-registration healthcare education programmes are three years long. Table 15.1 suggests how content about dignity can be sequenced across a three-year nursing programme; this sequence could be applied to other healthcare programmes. For trainee assistant practitioners and healthcare support workers, the timescale is shorter but the sequence of content in Box 15.2 is still applicable; the year 3 content could be reduced to take account of the different roles of these students. Dignity should be introduced early in the curriculum as this allows concepts to be developed and reflected upon as students grow in their professional role.

Table 15.1 Sample programme for dignity education

Year (when)	Content (what)	Method (how)	Rationale (why)
Year one			
Session 1	Explore dignity as a concept and relate it to practice	Reflective exercise as a trigger (*see* Reflective activity 15.2)	Exploration of personal concept
	What does the term 'dignity' mean to you?	Concept analysis – individual and then shared with other group members	Identification, sharing and comparing of elements that make up the concept
	What do the terms 'privacy', 'individuality', 'respect' mean to you?	Concept analysis – individual and then shared with other group members	Identification, sharing and comparing of meanings
	How do people show you respect? When are the times that you get privacy? What qualities and characteristics make you an individual?	Trigger questions; discussion	Identifies personal values
	What happens to dignity when someone is in need of nursing care?	Trigger question; discussion	Makes links to patients/ clients
	What actions can nurses take to maintain the person's dignity?	Trigger question; discussion	Links maintenance of dignity to professional role
	Person's view	Poem – *Crabbit Old Woman*	Appreciation of expert (patient's) view
Session 2	Policies; literature on empathy, compassion and caring – suggested articles given to the student	Directed reading and reflection	Opportunity for active engagement and for the student to formulate own ideas before sharing with fellow students
		Post on computer forum and comment constructively on peers' contributions	Group reflection may facilitate the presentation of alternative solutions and different interpretations of experiences but may suppress personal learning by leading to conformity (Jarvis, 1985, p.107). This is avoided by sharing after individual reflection. Places dignity in context with related values
Session 3	Appropriate attitude in relation to dignity	Trigger questions on verbal and non-verbal interactions, e.g. Do you say 'please' and 'thank you' to clients? Do you walk into a room/bed space before getting permission?	Students to relate these questions to themselves and decide on whether or not they are respectful

Year (when)	Content (what)	Method (how)	Rationale (why)
	Factors that influence the maintenance of patient dignity, e.g. gender, age, sexuality, disability, mental capacity	Reflection – identify groups of clients and an individual that the student has found easier to show respect to and less easy to show respect to	Consider factors that affect personal capacity to demonstrate respect. Compare personal factors to literature
		Discussion of literature on staff attitudes and equality and diversity	Consider the impact of experiences on self and how it shapes personal professional practice
	Promotion of choice	Trigger questions – list the choices that you have every week. Consider the choices that different client groups have in a week. How do they compare?	Consider the impact of experiences on self and how it shapes personal professional practice
	Promotion of privacy	Discussion on intrusion into own life and into clients' lives	
Year two			
Session 4	How dignity of clients can be maintained in student's own field of practice	User involvement – sharing their experience of dignity in healthcare and constructing a charter for dignity with the students	Gain client perspective
	Explore factors that could influence the maintenance of patient dignity and staff dignity in own field	Users to take the lead in formulating dignity charter, which students implement on placement	Experience the concept of partnership working and view the client as a colleague/ leader not a passive recipient
Session 5	Explore the concept of humanness and personhood	Experiential exercise, i.e. role play or simulation – sensory deprivation, disabled, homeless, confined to bed; or client/ family's narratives	First-hand experience of client situation. Not all students may wish to take part; or reflection on client/ family account
		Followed by reflective discussion on personhood. Bring in scenarios from other fields	Apply dignity to other fields
	Review charter from session 4	Discussion	Reflect on the experience of using the charter. Highlights barriers to and positive aspects of working for a client group

Table 15.1 continued

Year (when)	Content (what)	Method (how)	Rationale (why)
Year three			
Session 6	The emotionally vulnerable person	Trigger DVD followed by discussion and care planning	Taking time to 'see' what is happening for the patient during a time when there are clinical priorities that may be the staff's focus. Identifying actions that students can take to promote dignity
Session 7	The nurse's role in facilitating a culture that promotes dignity	Discussion on facilitating organisational culture. Reflective exercise (*see* Reflective activity 15.3). SWOB (strengths, weaknesses, opportunities, barriers) analysis of own ability to influence practice. Action planning – identify actions that the student will take to promote dignity – mini project on placement	To empower the students to influence the promotion of dignity in practice
	Dealing with challenging situations	Role play of challenging situations	To practise (through role play) relevant skills in a safe environment
Session 8	The nurse's role in facilitating a culture that promotes dignity	Feedback on the progress the student has made with his/her personal action plan	To review the impact the student has had on influencing promotion of dignity in practice – improving the service to patients
	Review and evaluate own practice		To enable the student to make the cognitive transition to qualified nurse

A detailed programme for dignity education in the university setting is outlined in Table 15.1. The programme would need to be linked to other educational sessions relating to values.

Selecting the how

A number of learning strategies can be considered when selecting the *how*. As previously discussed, strategies should adhere to the principles of deep learning, andragogy and constructive learning and some will aim to develop transformative learning. Examples of learning strategies include:

BOX 15.2 *Example of sequencing education about dignity in a three-year nursing programme*

First year: exploration of dignity as a concept and its relationship to practice
Two teacher contact sessions and one directed study
➤ Session 1: to take place before the first placement
➤ Session 2: directed study
➤ Session 3: to take place after placement experience

Second year: application of the concept to all fields of nursing
➤ Session 4: to take place in first half of year 2
➤ Session 5: to take place in second half of year 2

Third year: promoting dignity through influencing others
➤ Session 6: to take place in first half of year 3
➤ Session 7: to take place in first half of year 3
➤ Session 8: to take place in second half of year 3

➤ concept exploration (Fahrenwald *et al*, 2005; Vezeau, 2006; Vacek, 2009)
➤ use of triggers for discussion, for example, written scenarios, DVD, poetry, vignettes (Elfrink and Lutz, 1991; Gallagher, 2004; Shaw and Degazon, 2008)
➤ discussion/public dialogue/performance (Entwistle, 2000; Yorks and Sharoff, 2001; Warburton, 2003; Clare, 2007)
➤ narratives (Paterson and Crawford, 1994; Heliker, 2007; Cornwell and Goodrich, 2009; Trueland, 2009)
➤ reflection on practice including use of journals (Paterson and Crawford, 1994; Yorks and Sharoff, 2001; Lockyer *et al*, 2004; Chirema, 2006; Clare, 2007)
➤ role play (Shaw and Degazon, 2008; Cornwell and Goodrich, 2009)
➤ simulation (Elfrink and Lutz, 1991; Fahrenwald *et al*, 2005)
➤ role modelling and mentoring (Elfrink and Lutz, 1991; Paterson and Crawford, 1994; Stern, 2000; Weis and Schank, 2002; Illingworth, 2006; Peters, 2006; Vezeau, 2006; Armstrong, 2008; Cornwell and Goodrich, 2009)
➤ user involvement (Stuhlmiller, 2003; Clare, 2007; Morris and Faulk, 2007; Rush, 2008; Davison and Williams, 2009)
➤ action planning (Matiti *et al*, 2007).

Where should learning take place?

Some of the learning will occur in the formal education setting; other learning will occur in practice when the student is either trying out prior learning or being exposed to further new experiences. By far the majority of learning will need to take place in the student's own psychological space, if enduring and transformative learning is to occur.

Learning can occur in a range of physical environments: classroom, simulation, in a laboratory, or in practice. An environmental culture that promotes learning is pivotal to promoting dignity and it is the role of the teaching institution and individual teacher to promote a positive learning environment that enables deep learning to take place. This encompasses enthusiasm and empathy of the teacher (Entwistle, 2000), a caring and safe learning environment (MacNeil and Evans, 2005) and ensuring relevance of content and variation of teaching styles (Warburton, 2003) to take account of students' preferred learning styles, thus encouraging engagement with the topic. Entwistle (2000) cites Marton and Booth's (1997) idea of 'meetings of awareness': the teachers use their empathic awareness of what students already know and how they learn to develop their teaching strategies. Role modelling of nursing values by faculty staff forms a bridge between the environment and teaching strategies (Paterson and Crawford, 1994; Chou *et al*, 2003); for example, the teacher's willingness to accept a student's challenge to her opinion can lead to empowerment of the student – this willingness is an attribute of the teacher that will influence the culture of the environment and the strategies that will be used to teach.

Who is involved in promoting learning about dignity?

First and foremost, students themselves need to be receptive, active and reflective. Practitioners and service users have a large influence on students' learning too. Teaching staff have less opportunity in terms of time with students to facilitate learning; therefore, sessions need to be carefully planned to maximise their impact.

One learning strategy that illustrates how the questions of '*what, how, where, who* and *when*' form a useful framework is that of role modelling:

➤ *what* - according to the NMC (2007), student nurses should act as role models in promoting a professional image and in developing trusting relationships; therefore students are expected not only to become competent practitioners but to influence others

➤ *how* – can a person learn to be a role model? The evidence from the literature is that one learns to be a role model from another role model (Illingworth, 2006); this is particularly relevant to professionalism and values

➤ *where* – professionalism and values can be learned both in practice and in the academic setting

➤ *who* – in the practice setting, role modelling is learned from practitioners and the mentor has a key role (Armstrong, 2008); in the academic setting it is the responsibility of the educators (Paterson and Crawford, 1994) and other faculty staff. Peters (2006) discusses the value of educators in supporting students in clinical practice, thus bridging both settings

➤ *when* – role modelling of professionalism and values such as respect needs to be a continuous process; it cannot be switched on and off for a session if it is to be perceived as a genuine value of the role modeller.

Two Reflective activites (15.2 and 15.3) are included for you to consider – these form part of the sample programme in Table 15.1 (*see* sessions 1 and 7). These exercises will enable you to experience elements of the programme and evaluate their usefulness.

Reflective activity 15.2

You are attending an outpatients appointment for an examination and investigations due to recent rectal bleeding.

➤ What concerns do you have about the visit to the outpatients department?
➤ Does the thought of this appointment make you feel uncomfortable? If so, in what way?

You meet one of your neighbours in the waiting room – you know that, in the past, this neighbour has discussed other people's lives with other neighbours.

➤ What could the outpatient department staff do to prevent you feeling uncomfortable?

Reflective activity 15.3

➤ Identify one occasion when you maintained or promoted a person's dignity.
➤ Describe what you did.
➤ How do you know that this maintained/promoted this person's dignity?
➤ Why were you successful in maintaining/promoting this person's dignity?
➤ What can you take forward from this occasion to maintain/promote the dignity of others?

ASSESSMENT

Assessment has been suggested as a way of stimulating learning (Morris and Faulk, 2007). In a small qualitative study, ten students evaluated a range of assessments, including a community assessment, which involved assessing, planning, implementing and evaluating care outcomes from a holistic base and an individualised care planning assignment, and reported personal development in the value of human dignity (Morris and Faulk, 2007). Entwistle (2000) supports the use of assignments as a way of enabling students to demonstrate their understanding in an observable way. He also sees these 'performances of understanding' as an opportunity to develop the student's ability to think at a higher level. However, as previously discussed, formal assessment can impede deep learning and lead to what Entwistle (2000) terms 'an apathetic approach to study and surface learning'. To avoid this, the assessments need to be designed to reward personal understanding rather than reproducing knowledge. Formative rather than summative assessment will allow more freedom for the student to develop, as it reduces the fear of failing.

CONCLUSION

This chapter has emphasised the responsibility of universities to provide values education, incorporating dignity and respect. Other relevant values are integrity, empathy and compassion. It was argued that the ethical approach to teaching dignity should be most influential; however, the importance of both spirituality and politics was acknowledged. Application to practice is fundamental, as dignity education aims to improve the care experiences of service users. Due to the complexity and enduring nature of concepts that are part of a person's self-image, changes are difficult to effect. Therefore, education must provide opportunities for deep learning and facilitate learners in constructing their own meanings from their educational experiences in the university and practice environments. Only then can students transform their personal constructs and their professional practice. Educators must ensure that the environment is conducive to learning.

To be effective, theoretical educational approaches need to be translated into practical application. Kipling's five Ws and one H provide a useful framework for planning an educational programme. There are many learning strategies available; the final choice of strategy – *how* – for a session depends on the *what*, *when*, *where* and *who*. Role modelling was used as a bridge between concepts and application of theory. Assessment of learning is important to enable students to internalise their concept of dignity and transform their practice, thereby influencing others as a role model, as well as by explicit activities such as acting formally as an advocate. Summative assessment may impede internalisation and lead to surface learning; therefore, formative assessment may be more effective.

The chapter included a sample programme with suggestions for dignity education. As in any educational programme, the learning strategies used should be tailored to the learning styles of the students and the resources available. To conclude, deep learning and improving practice are fundamental in education for dignity in care.

ACKNOWLEDGEMENT

The authors would like to thank Mr R Brittle, lecturer, for his input to the questions in the sample programme for dignity education.

REFERENCES

American Association of Colleges of Nursing (1998) *The Baccalaureate: education for professional nursing practice.* Washington: American Association of Colleges of Nursing.

Armstrong N (2008) Role modelling in the clinical workplace. *British Journal of Midwifery* 16(9): 569–603.

Beattie V, Collins B, McInnes B (1997) Deep and surface learning: a simple or simplistic dichotomy? *Accounting Education* 6(1): 1–12.

Chirema KD (2006) The use of reflective journals in the promotion of reflection and learning in post-registration nursing students. *Nurse Education Today* 27: 192–202.

Chou S-M, Tang F-I, Teng Y-C *et al* (2003) Faculty's perceptions of humanistic teaching in nursing baccalaureate programs. *Journal of Nursing Research* 11(1): 57–63.

Clare B (2007) Promoting deep learning: a teaching, learning and assessment endeavour. *Social Work Education* 26(5): 433–46.

Cornwell J, Goodrich J (2009) Exploring how to enable compassionate care in hospital to improve patient experience. *Nursing Times* 105(15): 14–16.

Davison N, Williams K (2009) Compassion in nursing 2: factors that influence compassionate care in clinical practice. *Nursing Times* 105(37): 18–19.

Department of Health (2006) *Dignity in Care Public Survey October 2006. Report of the survey. Gateway number: 7213.* London: Department of Health.

Elfrink V, Lutz EM (1991) American Association of Colleges of Nursing essential values: national study of faculty perceptions, practices and plans. *Journal of Professional Nursing* 7(4): 239–45.

Entwistle N (2000) *Promoting Deep Learning Through Teaching and Assessment: conceptual frameworks and educational contexts.* Paper presented at the Teaching Learning Research Programme Conference, Leicester. www.tlrp.org/acadpub/Entwistle2000.pdf (accessed 13 October 2010)

Fagermoen MS (1997) Professional identity: values embedded in meaningful nursing practice. *Journal of Advanced Nursing* 25(3): 434–41.

Fahrenwald NL, Bassett SD, Tschetter L *et al* (2005) Teaching core nursing values. *Journal of Professional Nursing* 21(1): 46–51.

Gallagher A (2004) Dignity and respect for dignity – two key health professional values: implications for practice. *Nursing Ethics* 11(6): 587–99.

Heliker D (2007) Story sharing: restoring the reciprocity of caring in long-term care. *Journal of Psychosocial Nursing* **45**(7): 20–23.

Henschke JA, Cooper MK (2009) *International Research Foundation for Andragogy and the Implications for the Practice of Education with Adults*. www.umsl.edu/continuinged/education/mwr2p06/pdfs/B/Henschke_Cooper_International_research_foundation.pdf

Hoover J (2002) The personal and professional impact of undertaking an educational module on human caring. *Journal of Advanced Nursing* **37**(1): 79–86.

Human Rights Act. C.42. (1998) London: Her Majesty's Stationery Office.

Illingworth P (2006) Exploring mental health students' perceptions of role models. *British Journal of Nursing* **18**(13): 812–15.

Jacelon CS, Connelly TW, Brown R *et al* (2004) A concept analysis of dignity for older adults. *Journal of Advanced Nursing* **48**(1): 76–83.

Jarvis P (1985) *The Sociology of Adult and Continuing Education*. London: Croom Helm.

Jarvis P (1987) *Adult Learning in the Social Context*. London: Croom Helm.

Johnston MJ, Dacosta C, Turale S (2004) Registered and enrolled nurses' experiences of ethical issues in nursing practice. *Australian Journal of Advanced Nursing* **22**(1): 24–30.

Kalb KA, O'Connor-Von S (2007) Ethics education in advanced practice nursing: respect for human dignity. *Nursing Education Perspectives* **28**(4): 196–202.

Kipling R (1989) *Just So Stories for Little Children*. Harmondsworth: Penguin.

Lockyer J, Gondocz T, Thivierge RL (2004) Knowledge translation: the role and place of practice reflection. *Journal of Continuing Education in the Health Professions* **24**(1): 50–6.

MacNeil MS, Evans M (2005) The pedagogy of caring in nursing education. *International Journal of Human Caring* **9**(4): 45–51.

Manthey M (2008) Social justice and nursing: the key is respect. *Creative Nursing* **14**(2): 62–5.

Marton F, Saljo R (1976) On qualitative differences in learning. 1. Outcome and process. *British Journal of Educational Psychology* **46**(1): 4–11.

Matiti M (2002) *Patient Dignity in Nursing: a phenomenological study*. Unpublished PhD thesis. Huddersfield University.

Matiti M, Cotrel-Gibbons E, Teasdale K (2007) Promoting patient dignity in healthcare settings. *Nursing Standard* **21**(45): 46–52.

Mezirow J (2000) *Learning as Transformation*. San Francisco: Jossey Bass.

Morris AH, Faulk D (2007) Perspective transformation: enhancing the development of professionalism in RN-to BSN students. *Journal of Nurse Education* **46**(10): 445–51.

Nursing and Midwifery Council (2007) *Essential Skills Clusters for Pre-registration Nursing Programmes*. London: Nursing and Midwifery Council.

Pask G (1988) Learning strategies, teaching strategies and conceptual or learning style. In: Schmeck RR (ed) *Learning Strategies and Learning Styles*. New York: Plenum Press, pp.83–100.

Paterson B, Crawford M (1994) Caring in nursing education: an analysis. *Journal of Advanced Nursing* **19**(1): 164–73.

Peters MA (2006) Compassion: an investigation into the experience of nursing faculty. *International Journal for Human Caring* **10**(3): 38–46.

Quinn FM, Hughes SJ (2007) *Principles and Practice of Nurse Education* (5e). London: Croom Helm.

Raya A (1990) Can knowledge be promoted and values be ignored? Implications for nursing education. *Journal of Advanced Nursing* **15**(5): 504–509.

Rush B (2008) Mental health service user involvement in nurse education: a catalyst for transformative learning. *Journal of Mental Health* **17**(5): 531–42.

Sandberg J, Barnard Y (1997) Deep learning is difficult. *Instructional Science* **25**: 15–36.

Shaw HK, Degazon C (2008) Integrating the core professional values of nursing: a profession, not just a career. *Journal of Cultural Diversity* **15**(1): 44–50.

Social Care Institute for Excellence (2006) *Dignity in Care.* London: Social Care Institute for Excellence.

Stern DT (2000) The development of professional character in medical students. *Hastings Center Report* **30**(4): S26–9.

Stuhlmiller CM (2003) Breaking down the stigma of mental illness through an adventure camp: a collaborative education initiative. *Australian e-journal for the Advancement of Mental Health* **2**(2): 1–9.

Teeri S, Valimaki M, Katajisto J *et al* (2008) Maintenance of patients' integrity in long-term institutional care. *Nursing Ethics* **15**(4): 523–35.

Trueland J (2009) Compassion through human connection. *Nursing Standard* **23**(48): 19–21.

Tschudin V (2004) Editorial. *Nursing Ethics* **11**(6): 539–40.

Vacek JE (2009) Using a conceptual approach with concept mapping to promote critical thinking. *Journal of Nurse Education* **48**(1): 45–8.

Vezeau TM (2006) Teaching professional values in a BSN Program. *International Journal of Nursing Education Scholarship* **3**(1): 1–15.

Warburton K (2003) Deep learning and education for sustainability. *International Journal of Sustainability in Higher Education* **4**(1): 44–56.

Weinberg D, Weinberg GM (1983) Learning by design: constructing experiential learning programs. Proceedings of the Second Annual Information Systems Education Conference, 21–23 March, 1983, Chicago, USA.

Weis D, Schank MJ (2002) Professional values: key to professional development. *Journal of Professional Nursing* **18**(5): 271–5.

Williams B (2001) Developing critical reflection for professional practice through problem based learning. *Journal of Advanced Nursing* **34**(1): 27–34.

Woogara J (2005) Patients' rights to privacy and dignity in the NHS. *Nursing Standard* **19**(18): 33–7.

Yorks L, Sharoff L (2001) An extended epistemology for fostering transformative learning in holistic nursing education and practice. *Holistic Nursing Practice* **16**(1): 21–9.

CHAPTER 16

Enabling dignity in care through practice development

Kate Sanders and Jonathan Webster

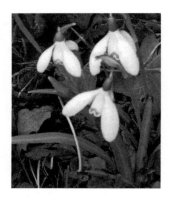

Awakening, whilst all around sleep,
icy cold encapsulates my world,
I persevere, I reach, I grow, I look upwards.
Light comes from my strength,
strength comes from my inner light.
I reach, I look upwards, I grow,
whilst all around awakens.

(Jonathan Webster)

INTRODUCTION

Defining dignity is complex; similarly, helping practitioners to develop practice (the ultimate aim being to improve the person's experience of care) in the context of complex work-based cultures and ever-changing services can be challenging. This chapter will consider how practice development can enable practitioners to improve dignity in care through creative, transformational ways of learning supported by skilled facilitation.

The first part of this chapter provides a brief history of practice development to set it into the context of the United Kingdom (UK) healthcare modernisation agenda. Practice development will then be defined and the key characteristics identified. Two pictures from practice describe how practice development can facilitate the development of people, practice and workplace cultures towards enabling the delivery of person-centred, evidence-based care. This chapter will also acknowledge some of the challenges within complex healthcare contexts and will identify core components that will help sustain and enable ongoing practice development.

LEARNING OUTCOMES

By the end of this chapter you will be able to:
➤ describe how practice development has emerged in the context of health-care modernisation
➤ identify the key concepts and methods of practice development
➤ recognise how practice development methods can be used to develop both practice and practitioners, to improve dignity in patient care
➤ understand some of the challenges of developing practice in complex workplace cultures.

PRACTICE DEVELOPMENT: A BRIEF HISTORY

Achieving and sustaining improvements in care is challenging, particularly when there is a constant drive to achieve economic efficiency and cost savings at all levels across organisations. It is therefore essential in our view that the workplace is receptive and open to ways of working that have improving quality at their core, but where staff feel empowered and enabled to think critically and work in new ways, the ultimate goal being to improve the quality of care for patients and for those people who support them.

Practice development has become a commonly used phrase to describe the variety of ways in which healthcare professionals develop their knowledge and skills to improve patient care (Titchen and Higgs, 2001; Garbett and McCormack, 2002; McCormack and Garbett, 2003; Manley and McCormack, 2004; McCormack et al, 2006) and that encompasses both nursing (Manley, 1997; McCormack et al, 1999) and the broader multiprofessional team (Walsh, 2000).

In order to understand the significance of practice development, it is useful to look at its emergence alongside other patient and healthcare developments.

In a recent review of the practice development literature, Shaw (2009) traces the development of practice development as a concept in the UK over the last three decades. She identifies the late 1970s as the starting point, with the move for nursing to become more patient centred through the introduction of the nursing process. This was followed by an increased emphasis on achieving quality healthcare through efficiency and productivity, which characterised the general management ideology of the 1980s (Griffiths, 1983), alongside which came further developments in nursing, including primary nursing (Pearson, 1983), nursing development units (NDUs) and, subsequently, practice development units (PDUs). Shaw (2009, p.24) suggests that the PDUs provided 'stepping stones toward the emergence of practice development as a concept', with the focus being on delivering patient-centred care that was of high quality and achieved through effective multidisciplinary working and a commitment to the development of nursing practice.

The 1990s saw an increased emphasis on the need for healthcare to be based on research evidence, which brought the concept of evidence-based practice to the fore (Shaw, 2009). However, the implementation of evidence into practice, for example via guidelines, is a complicated process (Royle and Blythe, 1998; Rycroft-Malone *et al*, 2002) and the assumption that once research and/or evidence is made available, it will be accessed by practitioners, appraised and then applied into practice is naïve (*Effective Healthcare Bulletin*, 1999) and often proves to be ineffective (Rycroft-Malone *et al*, 2002). Such findings suggest that alternative approaches to developing practice that take into account the complexities of healthcare practice contexts are needed.

The new British government in 1997 and their strong healthcare modernisation agenda could be seen as one of the most significant factors to support the emergence of practice development in the UK over recent years (McSherry and Warr, 2006). This agenda, supported by the introduction of new frameworks of accountability such as clinical governance, a variety of new roles, for example, practice development nurse, clinical practice facilitator, and new organisations such as NHS Quality Improvement Scotland and NHS Institute for Innovation to champion improvement in all four countries of the UK, has continued to be a major influence into the new millennium, with 'quality of care' as 'a central principle' being positioned alongside 'access, volume and cost of healthcare' (Royal College of Nursing, 2009).

Over the past ten years, there have been significant advances in the development of frameworks to guide practice development activities, and an increased understanding about the key underlying principles and methodological perspectives (McCormack *et al*, 2004; Manley *et al*, 2008). This work has been further strengthened by growing international collaboration, particularly between practitioners in the UK, Australia, New Zealand and Holland.

PRACTICE DEVELOPMENT: AN OVERVIEW

The term 'practice development' has frequently been used 'loosely' and interchangeably with others such as 'research into practice' (Mallett *et al*, 1997), and also to describe a broad range of educational (McKenna, 1995), continual professional development (Aggergaard *et al*, 2005; Walsgrove and Fulbrook, 2005), research (Rolfe, 1996) and audit (National Health Service Executive, 1996) activity. However, while in the past there has been a lack of clarity, a stronger and clearer understanding of practice development is emerging.

It can be argued that while practice development is directly concerned with the world of practice, if practice developers are to be effective, there is a need for them to be aware of and understand the assumptions that underpin the way that they work, and to use approaches that are systematic, rigorous and informed by their specific intended purposes (Manley and McCormack, 2004).

DEFINING PRACTICE DEVELOPMENT

The Department of Health (1993, 2003) has defined development (as in practice development) as a systematic process for change; however, Tolson *et al* (2006) argue that such a simplistic definition gives a false impression of the complexity of developing practice. A variety of more detailed definitions of practice development have been offered, and a summary of a selection (those based upon literature and/or contextually based evidence rather than opinion alone) is shown in Table 16.1.

These definitions help us to identify the key concepts of practice development, as they suggest both the purpose of practice development as well as the means by which this purpose is achieved. In summary, these definitions suggest that the purpose of practice development is improvement in healthcare, towards the achievement of effective and good-quality patient-centred care. The means by which this purpose is achieved have become increasingly refined but essentially include facilitation, the development of knowledge and skills, the use of processes that are systematic and rigorous and the transformation of contexts and cultures of care. It is argued that these activities need to be directly targeted at practice to have an impact on how practitioners work with patients, as opposed to just focusing on personal and/or professional development, which may or may not directly impact on practice (Manley and McCormack, 2004). Shaw (2009, p.63) argues that it is 'the emphasis practice development places on patients, their needs and their care that makes it distinct and arguably more effective in transforming practitioners and their practice.'

Practice development has, on occasions, been presented as a 'linear' or 'simple' educational process; however, there is increasing recognition that it is much more 'complex' and 'multifaceted' (Dewing and Wright, 2003). This complexity is articulated in an 'emancipatory' methodology of practice development (Manley and McCormack, 2004), which uses the concepts of critical social theory and emphasises the development of individual practitioners and the cultures and contexts within which they work to achieve sustainable changes in practice. This methodology is further refined in a recent revision of the McCormack and Garbett (2000) definition of practice development, proposed by Manley *et al* (2008) following critical dialogue with members of the International Practice Development Colloquium (a cooperative inquiry of practice developers, practitioner researchers and educators). It proposes that:

> Practice development is a continuous process of developing person-centred cultures. It is enabled by facilitators who authentically engage with individuals and teams to blend personal qualities and creative imagination with practice skills and practice wisdom. The learning that occurs brings about transformations of individual and team practices. This is sustained by embedding both processes and outcomes in corporate strategy (Manley *et al*, 2008, p.9, reproduced with permission from Wiley-Blackwell).

Table 16.1 Definitions of practice development

Author(s)	Definition of practice development	Informed by
Kitson (1994, p.5)	Practice development: • is a 'system' for introducing 'new activities or practices' • involves 'change agents' who 'work with staff' • is based on research, experience or 'trying out new ideas' • should be 'systematic' and 'carefully evaluated'	This definition emerged from nursing research and development activity supported by the National Institute for Nursing in Oxford
Mallett *et al* (1997, p.38)	Practice development is: • a 'continuous process' • linked to but different from professional development • concerned with using 'knowledge, skills and values' (professional development) to 'provide good-quality patient-focused care'	Mallett *et al* (1997) conducted a pilot study to explore the nature of professional development and practice development roles using questionnaires with nurses who were part of a professional and practice development nurses' forum
Unsworth (2000, p.323)	Practice development: • requires practitioners with multiple skills • introduces 'new ways of working' • is concerned with improving care or services • is concerned with sustaining or developing services • introduces changes that respond to client needs • results in effective services	These critical attributes of practice development were identified through the process of concept analysis, which was informed by dictionary definitions and literature
Garbett and McCormack (2002, p.88)	Practice development: • is a 'continuous process of improvement' • focuses on increasing 'effectiveness in patient-centred care' • focuses on achieving changes that reflect the perspective of service users • transforms cultures and contexts of care • is enabled by facilitation • uses 'systematic' and 'rigorous' processes	This definition emerged from a concept analysis, which was informed by literature analysis, telephone interviews and focus groups

This latest definition proposes that the purpose of practice development is the development of person-centred cultures, and places greater emphasis on the role of facilitation and the use of creativity (which has grown from the theoretical and methodological work of McCormack and Titchen [2006]) as the means for achieving transformations. This definition also highlights the importance of ensuring that practice development is not only embedded in practice but forms part of a strategic, corporate focus that will enable ongoing and active support for individuals and teams at a 'high level' within an organisation.

How is practice development approached?

Much of the success of practice development can be attributed to the way it is approached, and the connection between this and its outcomes for practice (Shaw, 2009).

A review of the evidence around practice development published in 2006 recommended that all practice development work should have evidence of a 'participatory, inclusive and collaborative methodology being used' (McCormack *et al*, 2006, p.11). In addition, 18 methods were identified that practice development projects should be able to demonstrate using. These methods have been themed by Shaw (2009, p.88; *see* Box 16.1), who suggests that an effective practice development project would emphasise each of six areas of significance.

Practice development or service improvement?

We have already acknowledged that the need to continuously improve the quality of care provided in the NHS is at the core of the UK government's programme for health service modernisation. It could be argued, however, that it is service improvement not practice development that has been embraced as a means of achieving these reforms. So what is the difference between practice development and service improvement?

Henderson and McKillop (2008) and Shaw (2009) have taken a closer look at the two concepts and acknowledge the similarities. They identify that both are concerned with improving patient care and use systematic and rigorous processes of change that are enabled by facilitators. Additionally, they both support the involvement of service users and other stakeholders; joint working across all healthcare services and settings; patient-centred care; and learning in and from practice. However, Henderson and McKillop (2008, p.339) believe that although there are many similarities between ideas and approaches, there are significant differences in the methods and the tools that are used. To summarise, service improvement largely focuses on 'systems and processes', while practice development concentrates on 'people and their practices.'

BOX 16.1 *Eighteen essential processes or methods for practice development identified by McCormack et al (2006) and themed by Shaw (2009) into six areas of significance*

1. Person-centred care
➤ Agreed ethical processes – 1
➤ Stakeholder analysis and agreed ways of engaging stakeholders – 2
➤ Person-centredness – 3

2. Collaboration and partnership
➤ Agreed ethical processes – 1
➤ Stakeholder analysis and agreed ways of engaging stakeholders – 2
➤ Person centredness – 3
➤ Values clarification – 4
➤ Developing a shared vision – 5
➤ Collaboration and participation – 7
➤ Developing shared ownership – 8

3. Enabling facilitation and support
➤ Methods to facilitate critical reflection – 10
➤ High challenge and high support – 11
➤ Facilitation of transitions – 15

4. Commitment to active learning and development
➤ Reflective learning – 9
➤ Methods to facilitate critical reflection – 10
➤ High challenge and high support – 11
➤ Feedback – 12
➤ Knowledge use – 13
➤ Giving space for ideas to flourish – 16
➤ Dissemination of learning – 17

5. Transforming workplace culture
➤ Workplace culture analysis – 6
➤ Rewarding success – 18

6. Evaluation
➤ Process and outcome evaluation – 14
➤ Dissemination of learning – 17

While there is a growing body of evidence to demonstrate the valuable contribution of service improvement to healthcare service development (Henderson and McKillop, 2008), Shaw (2009, p.301) argues that the use of practice development methodology 'could strengthen service development activity and increase participation in and sustainability of healthcare service improvement initiatives'.

PRACTICE DEVELOPMENT AND DIGNITY: 'PICTURES OF PRACTICE'

Picture one

This programme of practice development has been published (Webster *et al*, 2009) and presented at several conferences (Partners in Practice – University College London Hospitals NHS Foundation Trust 2008; International Practice Development Conference, Koningshof, The Netherlands 2008; Royal College of Nursing – Nursing Older People Conference, Manchester 2009).

Background

The profile and importance of dignity as a core component of essential care and a fundamental human right have attracted much attention. Different authors have identified the challenges of defining what is meant by 'dignity' (Fenton and Mitchell, 2002; Webster and Byrne, 2004; RCN, 2008); how patients (people) experience dignified or undignified care (Calnan *et al*, 2003; Woolhead *et al*, 2004; Age Concern, 2006) and the impact on person-centred outcomes and therapeutic relationships. In addition, sustaining and embedding dignity in how both individuals and teams work with older people remain challenging (Webster, 2007a).

Within the NHS trust in which this programme of practice development ran, I (Jonathan Webster), as consultant nurse for older people, had been asked to take a trust-wide lead in raising the profile of the importance of dignity in care at a time when there had been much publicity concerning the role of the 'dignity nurse' (Womack, 2006). This didn't mean that care within the trust was not dignified but rather that there was a need to make explicit the importance of dignity and to raise the profile of the importance of dignity and respect as part of all activities that involved patients.

I recognised how easy it was to espouse the importance and value of dignity in care (who wouldn't say that dignity is important?); however, more important, in my view, was the need to help staff embed change in clinical practice, to promote critical reflection leading to better understanding and insight, the core goal being to improve the patient's (person's) experience of care. While teaching, training and awareness raising play an important part in technical learning, I recognised that this was only a small part of the approach needed to enable change to occur (when it is needed) in highly complex and challenging work-based cultures and settings. As a nurse working with older people, practice development has played an important part in how I have worked with both individuals and teams (Webster, 2007b) in a number of different posts and organisations; the ultimate aim is to help individuals transform the way in which they work with patients and provide care, through skilled facilitation and work-based support.

Synopsis of the programme of practice development

The programme of practice development (reported in full by Webster *et al*, 2009) that ran for six months brought eight nurses and eight older people together to explore the meaning and understanding of dignity in care, using a variety of creative approaches such as collage and dance. Supporting each of the facilitated sessions was a reflective learning group for the nurse participants.

At the end of the programme, the nurses described how they had led changes in their clinical settings aimed at improving and raising the profile of dignity in care. These included improving methods of communication across the multiprofessional team; introducing preoperative visits to assess and meet patients; and the introduction of music to the clinical setting as part of the hospitals arts programme. Additionally, participants (both nurses and older people) described how the programme had not only raised their awareness but had enabled them to learn and share in an open, supportive environment. One older person stated:

> The discussions allowed me to open up and share experiences which have not been expressed before. I was comfortable but glad to get rid of the pain. The relief was immense.

Eloise (one of the nurse participants) described her experience of taking part and completing the programme (*see* Box 16.2).

Reflections/critique on learning

Throughout the programme of practice development the '18 essential processes or methods for practice development', as identified by McCormack *et al* (2006) and themed by Shaw (2009) earlier in the chapter, were evident at different times and stages of the journey.

This programme of practice development was not without its challenges. The real world of clinical care can be a highly challenging setting in which to work with practitioners, not only because of the day-to-day pressures of delivering services but also because of the broader influences asserted by both the work-based and organisational culture, which can be either enabling or disen-

BOX 16.2 *Vignette 1: Eloise*

This type of learning was very new to all of us. As nurses we were all used to the conventional teaching in a classroom where the teacher (the main focus) told you what you need to know, while in the approach taken with us as part of the programme we were teachers to each other, reflecting out loud or through the creative arts on good and bad practice. This allowed each of us to reflect on our own and with other group members' experiences. I wanted to immediately go straight back to the ward and share with my colleagues the type of 'care' patients are exposed to that compromises dignity, and to find out how our patients felt and from there how to change practice. This type of learning was very real; we saw group members' facial expressions of hurt, the pain in their eyes, when they had to share what had happened, and it reaffirmed (if there was any doubt) what a privilege it is, that people allow us as nurses, into their personal space at some of the hardest times in their lives. What became clear hearing people's stories was that what makes people feel respected is ensuring that care is given in a safe place, to be nursed by caring staff who will deliver individual patient centred care in a respectful, sensitive manner.

At the start of the programme we (the nurses and older people) were sitting at opposite sides of the room but by the end of the sessions we were working together and focused on making a difference to improve experiences of dignity. What was highlighted from the sessions was that everyone had their own meaning of dignity, but we all share the same idea that it is a fundamental human right and should be implicit as part of providing care. We each made our own objectives and plans of changing practice to bring back to our wards.

Within my own ward, a colleague and I set up a noticeboard where we could put up our names to highlight our roles to patients, families and staff as dignity champions, and also put up-to-date information on dignity in care and a suggestion box with comment cards to be filled in by patients during their stay so that they could tell us about their experiences of dignity in care on the ward. We recognised from listening to older people who took part in the programme that the environment in which care is delivered is important; rooms are now checked regularly to ensure curtains are fitted perfectly around the beds. Also we encouraged patients to wear their own night and day clothes and explained to patients and families the importance of upholding the rest period. On our wards the rooms are mostly single, so lack of privacy may not always be an issue but isolation and loneliness is a problem (this is something I had never thought about); plans are under way for a day room to be opened on the ward to enable patients to mix (if they wish) and to be able to eat away from the bedside too.

It is crucial in my area of practice (cardiothoracic surgery) to understand the complexities of caring for older people, as thoracic and cardiac surgery is invasive, and is being carried out increasingly on older people. It is essential for them to be supported and fully informed from admission to aftercare, as it will encourage faster recovery and enhance the experience of care. The next step for me is to translate my understanding of the importance of dignity in care into the clinical setting in which I work to help raise awareness in staff of the importance of dignified care. Even though this was a pilot programme of practice development, it would be so beneficial for all areas and teams to reflect and learn in a similar way, as the approach taken has transformed both my understanding and how I work as a nurse, which in turn has transformed care and raised the profile of the importance of dignity within the team in which I work.

Included with the permission of Eloise Horgan, Staff Nurse, University College London Hospitals NHS Foundation Trust.

abling to developing practice and new ways of working when there are competing pressures.

Through the sharing of stories based on reflection on action, nurse participants described how they were using the knowledge gained from the programme and their learning/collaboration with older people to influence how they worked with older people in their clinical settings on a day-to-day basis, with a clear focus on developing a greater person-centred approach to care. Conversely, through reflection, participants also described how they were increasingly reflecting in action when working with older people, and making sense of situations that they were facing.

Through facilitation (as part of the programme for nurses and older people) and group reflective learning for nurse participants, there was also evidence of group members increasingly challenging each other and their assumptions, beliefs and current ways of working. Such 'high challenge' required 'high support' to enable learning and better insight into their practice and the development of a shared understanding and, in turn, a shared vision. In the early stages of the programme, the majority of 'challenge' was provided by the older people as they shared stories and reflections of care; however, as the programme developed, nurse participants increasingly challenged each other and themselves, leading to a transition in both their understanding and how they practised.

Nurse participants described the importance of disseminating learning/knowledge and the need to help their colleagues to find both space and time to critically reflect on their own practice and to develop new ideas. Leadership and support in practice played a key role in enabling participants to 'grow', to carry the dignity agenda forward in their clinical setting and to 'own' developments. The ward sisters/charge nurses shaped this agenda and I observed that where developing practice and care was central to how the team worked and the work-based culture, the themes from the programme were more readily embraced by the team as a whole and applied to day-to-day practice with older people. More broadly, this also highlighted that the 'unseen' power of culture and the place of tradition and ritual should not be underestimated when helping practitioners to explore and critically question their practice. It appeared that for those nurse participants who were working in less 'receptive' work-based cultures, their need for support was greater as they tried to influence colleagues, peers and more senior staff.

Picture two

> The person with dementia is an individual with feelings – treat them with respect and dignity (Alzheimer's Disease International, 2009).

The purpose of this practice development initiative was to improve dignity in care for patients with dementia on an acute orthopaedic ward. It arose from concerns of senior nursing staff who had observed some of their nursing team delivering care that disregarded the older person involved, as they were focusing on achieving a task rather than the needs, desires or wants of the patient, causing distress for the patients and their families. Through discussions with the staff involved, and more general conversations with the clinical teams, it became apparent that development directly targeted at practice was needed to enhance staff awareness and understanding of the concept of dignity from the perspective of patients with dementia.

There were three key elements to this practice development initiative:

➤ three workshop days held in the hospital education centre facilitated by a clinical specialist in dementia care
➤ the development of a designated bay allocated for trauma patients with dementia called the 'forget me not' bay
➤ the creation of a working group of 'forget me not champions' to facilitate the exchange of ideas and implementation of actions to improve the hospital experience for this group of patients.

The world of practice – enhancing understanding of dementia and maintaining dignity

Following discussions with the senior nursing team, a workshop programme was developed and delivered by an external facilitator with expertise in dementia care and practice development. The workshop activities were targeted at practice, reflecting on and working with real clinical situations surrounding person-centred dementia care. The workshop was run on three occasions to enable day, night and therapy staff to attend. The involvement of as many staff as possible was seen to be essential, so that, collectively, they could explore and challenge current practice and develop a shared understanding of how care should be delivered and experienced.

Enhancing the environment

Practical and environmental measures can be taken to help support patients with dementia in the acute setting (Archibald, 2002). To achieve this, a six-bedded bay was designated for female patients with dementia. Using charitable funds, the room was decorated and furnished to provide a homely atmosphere with a sense of calm and with noise from the clinical unit reduced. Personal care plans have been introduced to enable staff to learn more about the patient and to enable them to communicate their likes, dislikes, needs and wants. Relatives are encouraged to provide information for the care plans and to bring in personal and familiar belongings for the patient. The introduction of open visiting has also enabled relatives to have greater involvement in care.

Stimulating and sustaining change

Staff were invited to form a working group to support the ongoing development of practice relating to dignity in care for patients with dementia. Twelve members of the multidisciplinary team now meet regularly to discuss issues, exchange ideas and reflect on how they can lead and facilitate new ways of working to continuously improve care. The demands of the unit are such that nursing time is precious, and so these meetings are short, but remain vital to ensure ongoing critique and to maintain motivation and enthusiasm.

Evaluating the impact

At a variety of stages through the process, staff and relatives were asked for their views and perspectives on how the workshops and environmental changes had impacted on the way in which care was delivered and experienced. This included the use of group reflection, written reflections and questionnaires. The following examples illustrate the ways in which staff believed that their knowledge and understanding of dementia had improved and how, as a result, the care they are giving has become more dignified, with greater emphasis on taking time and listening to the patients' needs and wants (also *see* Box 16.3).

I am now able to approach patients with an altogether new awareness of how they may perceive the environment around them.

I will no longer think of the job that has to be done. I will now look at the patient and wonder what they would like. I will listen more.

I enjoy working in the "forget me not bay". The focus of care is different. I can really relate to the patients and concentrate on what they need and what is going on.

When a patient is upset, angry and aggressive, I now try and see it from their point of view, be on their side and try and help them sort out the problem, or leave them alone if that's what they want. I used to ignore these emotions and carry on regardless, as I wanted to get the care delivery done. Now I wait until the patient is ready and in a state of well-being.

Relatives also reported positive experiences of care by the patients.

I feel you understand what my mother needs. I like the friendly atmosphere. It feels welcoming in here. I like the lights, pictures and music.

Thank you for letting me be involved in the care of my Mum. I like to be included and I always feel welcome. I like to help, and I know how busy you all are. This room has a special feel, and am pleased you make meal times and feeding an important issue.

Reflection on processes

The purpose of practice development as identified earlier in the chapter is continuous development towards the delivery of care that is person centred, and this picture from practice has demonstrated how this can be achieved for older people with dementia.

Within the context of therapeutic working with older people, Pritchard (2002, p.28) describes practice development as: '. . . helping practitioners within their real world context . . . to find creative and positive ways forward through the demanding, often confusing and draining day-to-day trials and tribulations of practice'. This view highlights the 'helping' and 'facilitative' approach needed by practice developers to work creatively with practitioners to help them to critically explore, and in doing so develop their practice at times when there may be immense pressure, or delivery of the 'quality' agenda may be difficult to achieve (Pugh *et al*, 2005).

Similarly, recognising that practice development's key aim is to 'improve' the person's experience of care, Hamer (2002, p.66) states: 'If practice devel-

BOX 16.3 *Vignette 2: Nikki*

Patient care is now delivered in a calm, quiet and relaxed atmosphere. Patients' personal needs are assessed and delivered in a timely and patient-focused manner according to what the individual wants. Ward routine is not adhered to in the bay and personal care is given as and when the patient needs. This is supported by personal care plans, which contain details of the patient's personal life stories, likes and dislikes.

The culture has shifted hugely. We are slowly becoming well known in the trust for delivering optimal and dignified care for this group of patients. The team are proud of the 'forget me not bay', and this sense of pride is reinforced by the positive feedback that we are constantly receiving from relatives and members of the multidisciplinary team. It is now a common conversation within the team to discuss individual patients and how we can meet their personal needs, however difficult this may be. The approach now is not how to get the job done but how can we make this as pleasurable as possible for the patient – going with the patient's flow and mood rather than a list of tasks. We enjoy their company and the bay has its own atmosphere and feeling.

At the beginning the staff strongly opposed the idea. New things were often met with suspicion and it was felt that the work load would be greatly increased as this group of patients had a poor status within the ward, as they were generally considered to be difficult and demanding to care for. From my perspective, there was an obvious lack of knowledge and understanding about dementia amongst staff. The workshop days were therefore really important in enabling change. The learning opportunities helped staff to develop an insight into the illness and to discover the ways in which they could meet the needs of patients and ensure that their experience of care was dignified and stress free. This involved exploring how to enter the patients' perspective and not to impose our reality. The 'forget me not champions' provided visible leadership and also helped to motivate the team.

With hindsight, I should have involved higher management more throughout the development to enable the initiative to have become trust-wide.

Included with the permission of Nikki Haak, Ward Manager, Royal Surrey County Hospital NHS Foundation Trust.

opment is a patient centred rather than a professional centred activity, as we believe it must be, then the extent to which we are able to gain insight into the perspective of service users, their perceptions, needs, wants and expectations, must be key to our success in this field'.

It is evident that skilled facilitation and transformational leadership have been fundamental to enabling this nursing team to critically explore their current ways of working, develop a deeper understanding of the patients' perspectives and consequently effect changes in the ways in which care is delivered and experienced. The culture of care within the 'forget me not bay' is now one that is centred on the needs and wants of the patients.

While it was senior staff who initially recognised the need for change, the processes used in this development enabled the multidisciplinary team to work collaboratively to achieve a shared understanding of how care should be delivered and experienced and to take ownership of the necessary changes to practice and the environment. Active involvement of relatives continues to enhance the person-centred approaches to care. The 'forget me not champions' and meetings provide ongoing critique and commitment to care and provide the time and space for new ideas to flourish.

While this project focused on enhancing dignity in care for patients with dementia, it would be interesting to explore how the methods used have impacted on dignity in care for patients on the ward who do not have dementia, as practice development is an approach that enables practitioners to work in person-centred ways regardless of the focus of care (Manley *et al*, 2008). Additionally, the need for active support from senior management and organisational strategy is recognised to enable the spreading, sharing and sustaining of good practice.

CONCLUSION

In healthcare today, traditional methods of integrating research and practice have been problematic, probably as a result of failing to recognise the complexity of the practice setting (Page and Hamer, 2002) and the competing pressures faced by practitioners and managers to deliver 'quality services' within strict financial constraints at times of immense change. Balanced against this is the need to recognise the requirement for sustained and systematic approaches to changing cultures of practice, in which we move beyond traditional notions of respecting and acknowledging individuality, and individualised care, to being person centred. Practice development has much to offer in meeting these competing demands.

At the start of this chapter, we identified that defining what is meant by 'dignity' is complex; similarly, helping practitioners to develop and change practice can be 'challenging' when the work-based culture is not supportive or open to enabling transformation in practice to occur. Embedding dignity and respect in the way in which practitioners work with patients and their supporters is core to delivering quality-focused services. However, we know that this can be problematic, as illustrated in a number of high-profile publications underpinned by harrowing stories when dignity has been diminished. Balanced against such harrowing stories and examples of undignified practice is the need to recognise in equal measure examples of practice where dignity and respect are core to how teams work and fundamental to how patients experience care.

We would argue that simplistic approaches to understanding complex phenomena such as 'dignity', 'clinical practice' and 'culture' will invariably lead to limited (if any) successful, sustainable improved outcomes for patients. In our view, both understanding and being able to work with complex work-based cultures are key to enabling the development of effective, person-centred practice. However, this doesn't happen haphazardly, it requires leadership, skilled facilitation and an approach to practice development that enables transformational change to occur and be sustained.

ACKNOWLEDGEMENTS

Eloise Horgan, Staff Nurse, University College London Hospitals NHS Foundation Trust; Nikki Haak, Ward Manager, Royal Surrey County Hospital NHS Foundation Trust; Theresa Shaw, Chief Executive, Foundation of Nursing Studies.

REFERENCES

Age Concern (2006) *Hungry to be Heard. The scandal of malnourished older people in hospital*. London: Age Concern.

Aggergaard Larsen J, Maundrill R, Morgan J et al (2005) Practice development facilitation: an integrated strategic and clinical approach. *Practice Development in Healthcare* 4(3): 142–9.

Alzheimer's Disease International (2009) *Living With and Caring For a Person with Dementia*. www.alz.co.uk/carers/caring.html#dignity (accessed 14 October 2010).

Archibald C (2002) *People with Dementia in Acute Hospital Settings*. Stirling: Dementia Services Development Centre, University of Stirling.

Calnan M, Woolhead G, Dieppe P (2003) Courtesy entitles. *Health Service Journal* 113(5843): 30–1.

Department of Health (1993) *Report of the Taskforce on the Strategy for Research in Nursing, Midwifery and Health Visiting (The Webb Report)*. London: HMSO.

Department of Health (2003) *Report of the Taskforce on the Strategy for Research in Nursing, Midwifery and Health Visiting*. London: HMSO.

Dewing J, Wright J (2003) A practice development project for nurses working with older people. *Practice Development in Health Care* 2(1): 13–28.

Effective Healthcare Bulletin (1999) Getting evidence into practice. *Effective Healthcare Bulletin* 5(1): 1–16.

Fenton E, Mitchell T (2002) Growing old with dignity: a concept analysis. *Nursing Older People* **14**(4): 19–21.

Garbett R, McCormack B (2002) A concept analysis of practice development. *Nursing Times Research* **7**(2): 87–100.

Griffiths R (1983) *NHS Management Inquiry Report.* London: Department of Health and Social Security.

Hamer S (2002) Innovation in practice. *Practice Development in Health Care* **1**(2): 66.

Henderson L, McKillop S (2008) Using practice development approaches in the development of a managed clinical network. In: Manley K, McCormack B, Wilson V (eds) *International Practice Development in Nursing and Healthcare.* Oxford: Blackwell Publishing, pp.319–48.

Kitson A (1994) *Clinical Nursing Practice Development and Research Activity in the Oxford Region.* Oxford: Centre for Practice Development and Research, National Institute for Nursing.

Mallett J, Cathmoir D, Hughes P *et al* (1997) Forging new roles: professional and practice development. *Nursing Times* **93**(18): 38–9.

Manley K (1997) A conceptual framework for advanced practice: an action research project operationalising an advanced practitioner/consultant nurse role. *Journal of Clinical Nursing* **6**(3): 179–90.

Manley K, McCormack B (2004) Practice development: purpose, methodology, facilitation and evaluation. In: McCormack B, Manley K, Garbett R (eds) *Practice Development in Nursing.* Oxford: Blackwell Publishing, pp.33–50.

Manley K, McCormack B, Wilson V (2008) Introduction. In: Manley K, McCormack B, Wilson V (eds) *International Practice Development in Nursing and Healthcare.* Oxford: Blackwell Publishing, pp.1–16.

McCormack B, Garbett R (2000) *A Concept Analysis of Practice Development.* London: Royal College of Nursing.

McCormack B, Garbett R (2003) The meaning of practice development: evidence from the field. *Collegian* **10**(3): 13–16.

McCormack B, Titchen A (2006) Critical creativity: melding, exploding and blending. *Education Action Research* **14**(2): 239–66.

McCormack B, Manley K, Kitson A *et al* (1999) Towards practice development – a vision in reality or reality without vision. *Journal of Nursing Management* **7**(5): 255–64.

McCormack B, Manley K, Garbett R (2004) A clearer vision of practice development? In: McCormack B, Manley K, Garbett R (eds) *Practice Development in Nursing.* Oxford: Blackwell Publishing, pp.315–29.

McCormack B, Dewar B, Wright J *et al* (2006) *A Realist Synthesis of Evidence Relating to Practice Development: Final Report to the NHS Education for Scotland and NHS Quality Improvement Scotland.* Edinburgh: NHS Quality Improvement Scotland.

McKenna H (1995) Nursing skill mix substitutions and quality of care: an exploration of assumptions from the research literature. *Journal of Advanced Nursing* **21**(3): 452–59.

McSherry R, Warr J (2006) Practice development: confirming the existence of a knowledge base. *Practice Development in Healthcare* **5**(2): 55–79.

National Health Service Executive (1996) *Clinical Guidelines: using clinical guidelines to improve patient care within the NHS.* London: HMSO.

Page S, Hamer S (2002) Practice development – time to realize the potential. *Practice Development in Healthcare* **1**(1): 2–17.

Pearson A (1983) *The Clinical Nursing Unit.* London: Heinemann.

Pritchard E (2002) Practice development, trials and triumphs. *Nursing Older People* 14(5): 28.

Pugh E, Locky M, McSherry R *et al* (2005) Innovation in practice: creating order out of chaos. Towards excellence in practice. *Practice Development in Health Care* 3(3): 138–41.

Rolfe G (1996) *Closing the Theory–Practice Gap: a new paradigm for nursing.* Oxford: Butterworth-Heinemann.

Royal College of Nursing (2008) *Defending Dignity – Challenges and Opportunities for Nursing.* London: Royal College of Nursing.

Royal College of Nursing (2009) *Breaking Down Barriers, Driving up Standards. The role of the ward sister and charge nurse.* London: Royal College of Nursing.

Royle J, Blythe J (1998) Promoting research utilisation in nursing: the role of the individual, organisation and environment. *Evidence-based Nursing* 1: 71–2.

Rycroft-Malone J, Harvey G, Kitson A *et al* (2002) Getting evidence into practice: ingredients for change. *Nursing Standard* 16(37): 38–43.

Shaw T (2009) *A Qualitative Descriptive Exploration of the Experiences of Healthcare Practitioners Involved in Practice Development.* Unpublished NursD thesis. University of Nottingham.

Titchen A, Higgs J (2001) A dynamic framework for the enhancement of health professional practice in an uncertain world: the practice–knowledge interface. In: Higgs J, Titchen A (eds) *Practice Knowledge and Expertise in the Health Professions.* Oxford: Butterworth Heinemann, pp.215–25.

Tolson D, Schofield I, Booth J *et al* (2006) Constructing a new approach to developing evidence based practice with nurses and older people. *Worldviews on Evidence Based Nursing* 3(2): 62–72.

Unsworth J (2000) Practice development: a concept analysis. *Journal of Nursing Management* 8(6): 317–22.

Walsgrove H, Fulbrook P (2005) Advancing the clinical perspective: a practice development project to develop the nurse practitioner role in an acute hospital trust. *Journal of Clinical Nursing* 14(4): 444–55.

Walsh M (2000) Chaos, complexity and nursing. *Nursing Standard* 14(32): 39–42.

Webster J (2007a) We all need to challenge practices that do not value a person's right to dignity. *Nursing Times* 103(15): 10.

Webster J (2007b) *Person-centred Assessment with Older People. An Action Research Study to Explore Registered Nurses' Understanding of Person-centred Assessment within a Framework of Emancipatory Practice Development.* Unpublished PhD thesis. University of Portsmouth.

Webster J, Byrne S (2004) Strategies to enhance privacy and dignity in care for older people. *Nursing Times* 100(8): 38–40.

Webster J, Coats E, Noble G (2009) Enabling dignity in care through practice development with older people. *Practice Development in Healthcare* 8(1): 5–17.

Womack S (2006) *Dignity Nurse in Every Hospital.* www.telegraph.co.uk/news/uknews/1516209/Dignity-nurse-in-every-hospital.html

Woolhead G, Calnan M, Dieppe P *et al* (2004) Dignity in old age: what do older people in the United Kingdom think? *Age and Ageing* 33: 165–70.

CHAPTER 17

Dignity in care: the way forward

Lesley Baillie and Milika Ruth Matiti

INTRODUCTION

This book has explored the concept of dignity from various perspectives, the factors influencing dignity for people in different care settings, and how dignity can be promoted. The two previous chapters of this section explored ways of educating about dignity and developing practice, with illustrative examples. In this final chapter, we will highlight key messages about dignity in care from this book and some of the challenges in the promotion of dignity in care, linking back to previous chapters. We will then focus on the implications for management and education. Finally, we will review research conducted about dignity in healthcare and consider further research needed to continue to develop the body of knowledge about dignity in care. The emphasis in this final chapter is on the way forward, for promoting dignity in care across the healthcare sector.

LEARNING OUTCOMES

By the end of this chapter you will be able to:
➤ explain the key messages relating to dignity in the care of people across diverse settings
➤ analyse challenges facing healthcare professionals striving to promote dignity in care
➤ discuss implications for healthcare management and education in relation to dignity in care
➤ consider further research needed to support dignity in care in the future.

DIGNITY IN THE CARE OF PEOPLE ACROSS DIVERSE SETTINGS: KEY MESSAGES

We have established the importance of dignity in healthcare for patients and clients, whether they are in hospital or community, acutely ill or living with a long-term condition, and whether they are at the beginning or end of their lives. A commitment to the concept of human dignity (*see* Chapter 2) is an important starting point for healthcare as it follows that all health service users should be treated as valued human beings by the healthcare system as a whole, and by the staff who work within healthcare organisations.

While we acknowledge the inherent dignity of each person, there are other meanings of dignity identified in the literature (*see* Chapter 2), which can be diminished within a healthcare context: for example, 'social dignity' (Jacobson, 2007, 2009) and the dignity of personal identity (Nordenfelt, 2003). A person's sense of dignity may alter during the course of a day, being affected by their circumstances and surroundings and their interactions with other people. Human beings, when ill or during life-stage processes such as giving birth (*see* Chapter 8) or dying (*see* Chapter 10), may experience changes in themselves that can threaten their dignity. The healthcare setting (*see* Chapter 5), other people's behaviour (*see* Chapter 6), and treatments, investigations and care activities further influence patients' dignity. For example, the dignity of people with mental health problems (*see* Chapter 13) or learning disabilities (*see* Chapter 14) has been diminished by society's attitudes, the care environment and the way in which these individuals have been treated by staff responsible for their care. Many reports have uncovered breaches of dignity of patients in acute hospital settings, due to a combination of healthcare systems, ward culture, individual staff behaviour, poor staffing levels and lack of resources. Reports from the United Kingdom (UK) such as the Patients Association's (2009) *Patients . . . Not Numbers, People . . . Not Statistics* indicate that there is much to be done before all patients, particularly those who are most vulnerable, can feel confident that their dignity will be protected and promoted in healthcare.

In Section 2, the chapters focused on dignity in different care settings and for varied patient or client groups, exploring specific factors that may increase vulnerability to diminished dignity and how staff can promote dignity. This section also considered contextual factors, including in some instances (*see* Chapter 13, mental healthcare) the historical factors. Dignity is complex: there is no one 'solution' or one way of working that will necessarily protect each individual patient's dignity in every setting and at every moment of the day. All these are challenges that healthcare professionals face in practice.

CHALLENGES FACING HEALTHCARE PROFESSIONALS WHO STRIVE TO PROMOTE DIGNITY IN CARE

Healthcare workers should not assume that promoting the dignity of patients or clients is 'easy' all of the time. There are challenges involved in the process. We argue that healthcare organisations and healthcare professionals should recognise the challenges, and indeed barriers, to promoting dignity in today's healthcare settings. Only then can we address these issues, through our healthcare practice, management of staff and organisations, and education. Here we identify key challenges for the promotion of dignified care, with examples from this book's chapters.

Challenge 1: attitudes and behaviour of staff

Staff attitudes and behaviour have a major influence on patient and client dignity (*see* Chapter 6). While we could assume that those who choose to work within healthcare professions will believe in the dignity of human beings and act accordingly in the care of patients and clients, we know that we cannot take this for granted as UK reports suggest otherwise (*see* Healthcare Commission, 2007, 2009; Patients Association, 2009). The issue is not confined to the UK; Jacobson's (2009) research details violations of dignity in Canadian healthcare settings and almost all relate to staff behaviour: rudeness, indifference, condescension, disregard, dependence, intrusion, objectification, restriction, labelling, contempt, revulsion, deprivation and abjection.

Other chapters detailed how the attitudes of healthcare professionals can affect the dignity of patients in specific patient groups or in particular settings; some examples follow. Paula Reed in Chapter 7 points out that staff may overlook the dignity of children and babies and that adults are used to having control over this age group within society. Staff may not always listen to young children as they try to express their needs, and instead communicate with parents, rather than the whole family. In Chapter 9, Wilfred McSherry and Helen Coleman suggest that negative attitudes towards older people and ageing in society as a whole may spill into healthcare too and lead to behaviour that undermines older people's dignity. In Chapter 13, Gemma Stacey and Theodore Stickley highlight that clients in acute mental health settings may not feel that they are treated with dignity, and while some factors are related to the care environment, procedures conducted by staff in mental health settings, such as restraint, may undermine dignity.

The challenge is therefore that each individual healthcare worker must recognise the inherent importance of dignity for each human being no matter what their situation or health condition, and ensure that dignity is central to their treatment and care. Staff should therefore constantly examine their attitudes and behaviour towards other people through self-reflection, which is an essential prerequisite to promoting dignity.

Challenge 2: vulnerability of patients and clients

Many of this book's chapters identified that patients' specific health conditions may affect their dignity, and thus healthcare staff have the challenge of promoting the dignity of people who may not be feeling dignified due to their situation; some examples drawn from this book's chapters follow. In Chapter 11, Candice Pellett explores the vulnerabilities of patients cared for in the community, many of whom may have long-term debilitating conditions that affect their everyday life. Gemma Stacey and Theodore Stickley in Chapter 13 highlight that older people may have experienced years of mental health problems alongside associated social consequences, and older people with Alzheimer's disease can be both physically and mentally frail. In Chapter 12, Lesley Baillie highlights the particular vulnerability of patients in acute and critical care settings, as they often experience anxiety, fear, loss of control and dependency, and undergo procedures that are invasive, exposing and embarrassing. Patients could be unconscious, and undergo surgery or resuscitation; in such situations patients have no control over their bodies and are dependent on staff to promote their dignity. Furthermore, an individual's dignity may be affected by life stage; Paula Reed (Chapter 7) identifies particular dignity issues of different age groups. Young children and babies cannot always clearly identify their needs, and adolescents are undergoing considerable physical and emotional changes.

Challenge 3: the care environment

In the Royal College of Nursing's (RCN; 2008) nursing workforce survey, many respondents gave examples of how resource shortages (staff, space and equipment) affected delivery of dignified care. These factors may lead to staff feeling that their own dignity is diminished by their employing organisation, affecting their ability to promote patients' dignity. In Chapter 4, Alistair Hewison examines how healthcare staff are confronted by apparently conflicting priorities; they have time-driven targets to meet, which in turn impact on the patient care experience. Ann Gallagher's exploration of how the care environment affects patients' dignity (*see* Chapter 5) highlights aspects such as privacy and organisational culture. Kate Sanders and Jonathan Webster, in Chapter 16, discuss how practice developments in dignity are influenced by environmental culture. Other chapters provide specific examples of how the care environment can impinge on staff who are striving to promote dignity; here are some examples. In Chapter 7, Paula Reed discusses how lack of privacy affects children's dignity in hospital, as wards may have mixed age groups and the imposed mealtimes and other routines remove independence and control from children. In Chapter 12, Lesley Baillie details how the high workload of acute hospitals impacts on patients' dignity. She highlights that staff–patient relationships are affected by healthcare systems in acute care that lead to frequent transfers of patients. In Chapter 13, Gemma Stacey and Theodore Stickley explain how mental healthcare systems and care environments have encroached on the dignity of people with mental health problems.

These challenges all have implications for healthcare management and education.

THE IMPLICATIONS FOR HEALTHCARE MANAGEMENT

Managerial issues might relate to resources, systems and processes (for example, excessive patient transfers) and care environment concerns, as well as managing individual staff behaviour. The promotion of dignity in healthcare needs commitment from politicians and healthcare management authorities as well as individual healthcare organisations, such as hospitals, community services or care homes. It is evident in the literature that healthcare settings lack resources on a worldwide basis. There should be continuous lobbying of governments so that more resources are allocated to healthcare services because, without enough resources, it is difficult to promote dignity in healthcare, even for highly committed healthcare workers. However, healthcare workers should maximise the use of limited resources, which can be achieved better with improved knowledge, skills and appropriate attitudes and behaviour. In the UK, the Darzi report emphasised that organisations should 'organise care around the individual, meeting their needs not just clinically, but also in terms of dignity and respect' (DH, 2008, p.21). There are many managerial strategies in place already to facilitate dignity in care for patients and clients.

From a human resource dimension, wards need an adequate and stable workforce, with dignity-promoting leadership and a whole-ward culture and commitment to patient dignity. Healthcare organisations need to consider how they can recruit and select staff with appropriate attitudes and insights that will promote patient or client dignity. Staff recruited to work in healthcare must have insight into the reasons why patients may be vulnerable to their dignity being diminished, and display compassion for those whom they care for. They should want to do their best for patients, understand how to behave towards patients in a way that will promote dignity, and have a willingness to challenge dignity compromises. Therefore, we suggest that interviewers should explore understandings of dignity with applicants and set out an absolute expectation that all staff will behave towards patients in a way that promotes dignity. Box 17.1 suggests interview questions to use and the types of responses an interviewer would look for. Some organisations include service users in interview panels so that they can consider whether the interviewee is the type of person who they would like to care for them.

Once staff are employed, organisations should have strategies for supporting staff to promote the dignity of patients and clients. Managers should consider what type of policies and regulations they have in place to specifically address the dignity of patients and clients. For example, in the UK, the Department of Health's (DH) ten-point challenge for healthcare organisations (*see* Chapter 4) sets out expectations (DH, 2006a). There are NHS trusts that require all staff to sign a pledge that they will behave in accordance with the DH dignity challenge, thus setting a clear expectation that their staff will promote dignity in care. As discussed in previous chapters (*see* Chapters 1 and 3), registered healthcare professionals are required to behave according to their professional bodies' codes of conduct and ethics too, and can be called to account for their behaviour. Strong leadership for dignity is very important within healthcare

---

BOX 17.1 *Key questions to explore at interview*

➤ Why do you want to work for this organisation/study this course?
Look for: an interest in people and a desire to care for/help people who are undergoing healthcare.

➤ We expect all healthcare staff to behave towards patients in a way that promotes their dignity. Please give some examples of how you could promote dignity for patients. *Look for: communicating respectfully (for example, introducing yourself and addressing the person by their preferred name), treating people as individuals and as important and valued human beings, providing privacy, explaining and informing patients, being kind and compassionate.*

➤ Why might people (*individualise question to relevant client group, for example, children, older people, people with mental health problems or learning disabilities*) be vulnerable to a loss of dignity when undergoing healthcare? *Depending on the client group and setting, look for: loss of independence and control, fear and uncertainty, being undressed and undergoing procedures, lack of privacy.*

➤ What do you think could cause a lack of dignity for patients? *Look for: lack of privacy, staff behaving as though the patient does not matter by ignoring, talking down, being rude, disrespectful or unkind; lack of attention to fundamental human needs, such as hygiene, comfort and food.*

➤ What would you do if you thought a patient was being treated with a lack of dignity? *Look for actions to promote dignity, such as kindness and providing comfort and privacy, challenging the colleague, reporting to a senior colleague.*

---

organisations (*see* Chapter 5), and an ethos of dignity in care needs to pervade the whole organisation.

Organisations should create a culture that encourages feedback from staff and patients and have procedures to monitor dignity on an ongoing basis. There should also be clear and accessible procedures for reporting and dealing with dignity compromises. In England there are mandatory inspections for healthcare organisations (the Care Quality Commission, Patient Environment Action Team), which include criteria for dignity, respect and privacy. These inspections ensure that dignity and privacy are seen as important in organisations, as their ratings are published and no organisation would want to score badly on these aspects. However, the more qualitative aspects of a patient's healthcare experience are not easily measured in such quantitative terms (Picker Institute

2008), so organisations need to consider how they can gain more meaningful feedback from their local populations. The UK government recommends that trusts, clinical teams, professionals and commissioners develop their own quality indicators, tailored to local needs, specific conditions and specialties (Sizmur *et al*, 2009). Organisations should therefore work closely with their local service user groups to gain feedback and evaluate improvements made. Many organisations have their own systems for monitoring dignity, such as dignity audits and matrons' rounds. For example, in the RCN survey, a manager reported:

> We have a stop-and-look programme in which matrons walk the wards with staff of different grades and challenge them to look into patient bays and think whether, if their family members were there, they would be happy or confident about their care. This has made nurses really look at their practice and how their patients are treated (RCN, 2008, p.39, reproduced with permission from the Royal College of Nursing).

Some organisations use electronic patient experience trackers to measure patient and staff satisfaction at the point of delivery. These devices can be used to evaluate dignity and privacy issues, as well as any other aspect of patient experience, and they can instantly capture the patient's experience on a 24-hour basis, enabling timely feedback on any developments implemented to enhance care. Dewar *et al* (2010) described using 'emotional touch-points' to elicit patients' and relatives' views of their care from an emotional perspective. Patients and families are asked about key points in the patient's journey and they select emotional words (provided on cards) to portray how they felt at that point. Dewar *et al* (2010) argue that this method leads to a more balanced and meaningful representation of patients' care experiences. The findings were then used to improve compassionate care within an action research project.

In terms of care environments, as Ann Gallagher discussed in Chapter 5, there are fundamental aspects of the physical environment that are necessary to promote patients' dignity or at least to make it easier for staff to do so. Some factors relate to privacy, for example, single-sex accommodation, bed curtains that fit properly, bed spaces of adequate size and sufficient toilets and bathrooms. In England recently, the Design Council worked with the DH on a project called 'Design for Patient Dignity' which aimed to tackle environmental challenges to dignity (particularly privacy) from a design perspective (see www. designcouncil.org.uk). Other essential factors are environmental cleanliness and easy access to appropriate food for patients.

Healthcare organisations should have systems that treat patients as valued individuals. However, in the UK, bed shortages in some hospitals have led to the constant moving of patients between wards, and to patients being in mixed-sex accommodation (now being eliminated, *see* Chapter 4's discussion). Bed management systems should ensure single-sex environments and minimal transfers, and that patients with similar conditions are cared for together, thus promoting social support and mutual understanding (Baillie, 2009). For many patients, their relationships with staff and sometimes with other patients (Baillie, 2009; Bridges and Nugus, 2010) are important for their self-esteem and for feeling that they are cared for as individuals. Frequent moving of patients between wards disrupts relationships with both staff and other patients.

The dignity of healthcare workers is also important. The UK has a 'Dignity at Work' policy (*see* www.dignityatwork.org). The underlying assumption is that it is difficult to expect healthcare workers to think about patients' dignity if their own dignity is at stake. Watson (1996) claims that only if nurses treat themselves or are treated with dignity will they treat their patients or clients with respect, care, gentleness and dignity. In the RCN (2008) survey, nurses confirmed her view; for example, one hospital staff nurse said:

> My last shift only stopped for lunch at 4pm and I did not have time to have a drink with it. I did not have time to drink a hot drink from 10am to 6pm. I think nurses need to be treated with dignity if we are to deliver the same (RCN, 2008, p.31, reproduced with permission from the Royal College of Nursing).

In Chapter 5, Ann Gallagher considers how organisational culture influences dignity. Staff who appear uncaring could be suffering from burnout or may be exhausted and demoralised. Staff are human beings too, whose dignity can be threatened by circumstances and how others behave towards them, for example, inadequate resources to carry out their job, excessive workload and unsupportive colleagues and senior staff.

In England, under the auspices of the DH Dignity in Care campaign (DH, 2006a), many staff have signed up as dignity champions (*see* Chapter 4). In some organisations, there are dignity champions throughout the organisation. While any staff member can ensure that their own individual practice with patients promotes dignity, a group of dignity champions, recognised and supported by their organisation and with opportunities to share good dignity practices through forums, can make a much larger and more sustained impact on dignity within an organisation. Local dignity champions can work with their teams and patient groups to identify dignity issues and tackle these and develop dignity-promoting practice. In Chapter 16, Kate Sanders and Jonathan Webster explain how practice can be developed, including detailed examples of how a planned approach can lead to real differences being achieved. Crow *et al* (2010) established a 'dignity forum' in a hospital, in response to individuals feeling isolated in their efforts to enhance dignity.

IMPLICATIONS FOR EDUCATION OF HEALTHCARE WORKERS

Recruitment and selection, as discussed earlier (*see* Box 17.1), also apply to recruitment of healthcare students, so that educators can ensure that students recruited hold the fundamental values necessary to underpin care with dignity. We must then consider how healthcare education can further develop appropriate attitudes and from what base point. Dignity education should start in pre-registration programmes, as students are the future workforce of healthcare organisations. Patient dignity should be explicit and integral in pre-registration and postregistration healthcare courses, so that students can explore and understand the subject. Thus, curriculum teams must plan effective education to enable healthcare students to learn about dignity and apply their learning in practice. We suggest that curricula for healthcare students should be evaluated to see what, how, where and when dignity is being taught. In Chapter 15, Liz Cotrel-Gibbons and Milika Ruth Matiti detail approaches to education about dignity that can help to develop knowledge, skills and appropriate attitudes among healthcare students.

Healthcare settings need to have staff who understand the meaning of dignity, are vigilant about, and sensitive to, how the dignity of patients could be undermined, are committed to promoting dignity in care, and act as role models for dignified care in practice. Therefore, all staff with patient contact (including non-clinical staff such as receptionists) need education about patient dignity, as recognised by a number of writers (Lothian and Philp, 2001; Woogara, 2004a). As Alistair Hewison points out in Chapter 4, there are many sources of information available to practitioners to inform them about how to care for patients with dignity. The challenge is more about staff accessing and then applying this information in their practice. Healthcare workers need to acquire sound knowledge to underpin dignified care delivery and develop healthcare skills related to dignity in care. Staff also need to develop appropriate attitudes and values, as it is through attitudes that staff portray that the patient is valued (Bayer *et al*, 2005). Some staff may lack the specific knowledge to underpin behaviour that promotes dignity; for example, they may lack the knowledge and skills to care for people with specific needs, such as those with learning disabilities or a mental health problem. They could lack skills in fundamental care, for example, supporting patients with nutritional intake, pain management or end-of-life care. A lack of knowledge and skills may lead to inappropriate and unhelpful attitudes, avoidance of patients, or omissions in care. Therefore, staff must have further education about dignity, to ensure that they acquire the knowledge, skills and attitudes that underpin behaviour that promotes dignity in care. Education can also affirm the organisation's commitment to patient dignity and help staff to understand how to recognise and deal with any dignity compromises encountered.

Education should include service user involvement, as listening to and exploring patients' real experiences of dignity in care is meaningful and has a high impact. Patients' real experiences can be explored through digital story-telling and extracts from reports (for example, Patients Association, 2009 – *see* Chapter 9 as an example). Teaching methods should be active, with participants rehearsing interactions that promote dignity, and practising how they can provide privacy, in simulated care situations. Active learning promotes deep learning (*see* Chapter 15), which can be applied more readily in practice (Biggs, 1999). The teaching methods used need to trigger awareness of students' practice: how their own actions affect the dignity of patients and how their behaviour can influence their colleagues' behaviour. With every care activity or procedure healthcare students learn, the teaching of care with dignity should be integral, with facilitators asking, how might this procedure affect dignity and how can you protect dignity? Clinical staff education should give special consideration to promoting patients' dignity during intimate and invasive care and examinations. Healthcare students and employees need to develop awareness of their ethical and professional responsibilities to promote dignity (*see* Chapter 3), learn to take individual responsibility for patients' dignity and develop an understanding of how the impact of their own actions and omissions in care could affect the dignity of patients. They also need to learn to recognise and report factors that affect dignity, such as the care environment and resource issues, and consider how to address dignity compromises. Staff must therefore be educated about managing ethical dilemmas; the use of critical incidents and reflective practice can help staff to learn from their experiences.

As promoting dignity is a collective responsibility of all healthcare workers, all those involved in the patient or client journey in healthcare should have the opportunity of learning together through interprofessional education. Barr and Goosey (2002, p.2) cited a revised definition of interprofessional education for the Centre for the Advancement of Inter-professional Education (1997) as: 'when two or more professions learn, from and about each other to improve collaboration and quality of care'. Collaboration between different professions is important if quality care is to be achieved; therefore, students and staff from different professions need to learn together. It was evident from Matiti's (2002) study that some indignities to patients result from healthcare workers not understanding or appreciating other professionals' roles.

RESEARCH THAT WILL SUPPORT DIGNITY IN CARE IN THE FUTURE

Considering how important dignity is to patients and clients in every society, there is comparatively little research carried out worldwide. However, if a concept is important in clinical practice, then even limited study of the concept is useful (Chinn and Kramer, 1995). Studies have mainly focused on the meaning of dignity and factors affecting dignity in healthcare settings, while research about how dignity issues can be tackled, and the barriers to dignified care, are less apparent. Most studies have been conducted in the last decade, perhaps due to a greater awareness of the importance of patient experience and human rights as a whole, particularly in the UK. These studies are all important, in that they have made a contribution to the body of knowledge about patient dignity and they have raised awareness of the indignities that patients and clients face while receiving healthcare. Research has focused predominantly on hospital patients and adults. Few studies have considered community patients, children, women using maternity services, or people with mental health problems or learning disabilities.

Table 17.1 summarises designs and methods used to study dignity. Most studies have been qualitative, which is unsurprising, as qualitative research is more suited to studying human experiences, such as dignity.

Table 17.1 Research designs and methods used to study dignity

Design and methods	Researchers
Questionnaire survey	Matiti and Sharman, 1999; Rylance, 1999; Whitehead and Wheeler, 2008
Internet/online survey, including free-text answers	Gamlin, 1998; DH, 2006b; RCN, 2008
Rating scales	Hack *et al*, 2004
Phenomenology – interviews	Pokorny, 1989; Matiti, 2002; Walsh and Kowanko, 2002; Enes, 2003; Widäng and Fridlund, 2003; Öhlén, 2004; Widäng *et al*, 2008; Webster and Bryan, 2009
Ethnography – interviews and observation	Reed *et al*, 2003; Woogara, 2004a,b; Reed, 2007
Grounded theory – interviews/observation	Jacelon, 2003; Jacobson, 2009
Case study – observation, interviews, documentary analysis	Baillie, 2007; Baillie and Gallagher, 2010
Discourse analysis – interviews and documentary analysis	Street, 2001
Qualitative – interviews	Chochinov, 2002; Matthews and Callister, 2004; Bridges and Nugus, 2010; Slettebo *et al*, 2009
Quasi-experimental pilot study – observation, attitude measurement scales, interviews	Seedhouse and Gallagher, 2002
Focus groups	Stabell and Nåden, 2006; Bayer *et al*, 2005; Stratton and Tadd, 2005; Ariño-Blasco *et al*, 2005
Observation	Randers and Mattiasson, 2004; Lundqvist and Nilstun, 2007
Action research	Turnock and Kelleher, 2001; Crow *et al*, 2010

Most studies included patients and/or nurses as participants; only a few studies included interviews with relatives or carers (Seedhouse and Gallagher, 2002; Street, 2001; Jacelon, 2002, 2003; Enes, 2003; Bridges and Nugus, 2010). However, relatives of patients are often highly distressed by indignity (*see* Patients Association, 2009), and therefore exploring their views is very relevant. Many of the most vulnerable patients (for example, unconscious, dying, advanced dementia) are the most difficult to include in research due to access and consent issues, and they have therefore been excluded from studies. Including relatives of vulnerable patient groups in future research could be most insightful. Interviews with healthcare professionals other than nurses is noticeably absent, even though promoting dignity is an interprofessional activity.

Although a number of studies about dignity have been published, as discussed above, there is a need for further research in different settings and from different perspectives. We suggest that there should be research about how patients in different healthcare settings and in different countries perceive their dignity. Dignity is a cultural concept and it should be understood within the different contexts/organisational cultures. Intercultural research about the concept of patient dignity might provide a global operational definition. Furthermore, the healthcare setting's culture is continually changing and evolving due to developments such as technology. It is logical, therefore, to assume that perceptions of dignity will also change, necessitating updating of the concept. Practical ways of promoting dignity that are based on evidence should continue to be identified. More research on influencing factors such as the environment, attitude of patients and behaviours of different staff in different professions is also needed. Research to investigate gender influences on the dignity of patients or clients would provide useful insights. Action research studies, which would enable study of how practice might be changed, incorporating study of dignity-promoting organisational cultures, would make a valuable contribution too.

Although this book is primarily concerned with patient or client dignity, it is worth mentioning that research about the dignity of healthcare staff is very difficult to find. As discussed earlier, the dignity of healthcare workers needs to be upheld too, so that they in turn can effectively promote patient or client dignity. Researchers could explore the interrelationship between staff and patient dignity. It is also evident from the literature that there is a paucity of tools to evaluate dignity in practice.

CONCLUSION

Dignity in healthcare needs commitment at all levels, from government, healthcare organisations, teams and individual staff. Dignity must be tackled from an environmental and resource perspective but we also need healthcare staff who feel confident that they can make a difference to dignity in care and that their team, their organisation and managers will support them. While research studies about dignity have grown in number over the last decade, we have identified a number of gaps and suggested further areas for research. Findings from empirical studies should inform healthcare practice and policy and also inform healthcare curricula and influence how dignity in care should be taught. Healthcare workers must have the support of their organisations so that they can promote patients' dignity, and they should feel confident that their own dignity will be preserved at work.

All healthcare patients are vulnerable to their dignity being threatened; conversely, patients who feel that their dignity is promoted will have a better healthcare experience. Patients may have illnesses that cannot be cured and they may face an uncertain future and prognosis. They should always be able to be confident that they will be treated with dignity.

REFERENCES

Ariño-Blasco S, Tadd W, Boix-Ferrer JA (2005) Dignity and older people: the voice of professionals. *Quality in Ageing* 6(1): 30–5.

Baillie L (2007) *A Case Study of Patient Dignity in an Acute Hospital Setting.* Unpublished thesis. London South Bank University.

Baillie L (2009) Patient dignity in an acute hospital setting: a case study. *International Journal of Nursing Studies* 46: 22–36.

Baillie L, Gallagher A (2010) Evaluation of the Royal College of Nursing's 'Dignity at the heart of everything we do' campaign: exploring challenges and enablers. *Journal of Research in Nursing* 15(1): 15–28.

Barr H, Goosey D (2002) *Inter-Professional Education: selected case studies.* Commissioned by the Department of Health from the UK Centre for the Advancement of Inter-professional Education (CAIPE). www.dh.gov.uk/en/Publicationsandstatistics/Publications/PublicationsPolicyAndGuidance/DH_4139354

Bayer T, Tadd W, Krajcik S (2005) Dignity: the voice of older people. *Quality in Ageing* 6(1): 22–7.

Biggs JB (1999) *Teaching for Quality Learning at University.* Buckingham: Open University Press.

Bridges J, Nugus P (2010) Dignity and significance in urgent care. *Journal of Research in Nursing* 15(1): 43–53.

Centre for the Advancement of Inter-professional Education (1997) *Inter-Professional Education – A Definition.* London: Centre for the Advancement of Inter-professional Education.

Chinn PL, Kramer MK (1995) *Theory and Nursing – A Systematic Approach* (4e). London: Mosby.

Chochinov HM, Hack T, McClement S, Kristjanson L, Harlos M (2002) Dignity in the terminally ill: a developing empirical model. *Social Science and Medicine* 54(3): 433–43.

Crow J, Smith L, Keenan I (2010) Sustainability in an action research project: 5 years of a dignity and respect action group in a hospital setting. *Journal of Research in Nursing* **15**(1): 55–68.

Department of Health (2006a) *Dignity in Care*. Gateway reference 7388. London: Department of Health.

Department of Health (2006b) *Dignity in Care Public Survey October 2006 – Report of the Survey*. Gateway reference 7213. London: Department of Health.

Department of Health (2008) *High Quality Care For All – NHS Next Stage Review final report*. Gateway reference 10106. London: Department of Health.

Dewar B, Mackay R, Smith S, Pullin S, Tocher R (2010) Use of emotional touchpoints as a method of tapping into the experience of receiving compassionate care in a hospital setting. *Journal of Research in Nursing* **15**(1): 29–41.

Enes SPD (2003) An exploration of dignity in palliative care. *Palliative Medicine* **17**(3): 263–9.

Gamlin R (1998) An exploration of the meaning of dignity in palliative care. *European Journal of Palliative Care* **5**(6): 187–90.

Hack TF, Chockinov HM, Hassard T *et al* (2004) Defining dignity in terminally ill cancer patients: a factor-analytic approach. *Psycho-oncology* **13**: 700–708.

Healthcare Commission (2007) *Caring for Dignity: a national report on dignity in care for older people while in hospital*. London: Commission for Healthcare Audit and Inspection.

Healthcare Commission (2009) *Investigation into Mid Staffordshire Foundation Trust*. London: Commission for Healthcare Audit and Inspection.

Jacelon CS (2002) Attitudes and behaviours of hospital staff towards elders in an acute care setting. *Applied Nursing Research* **15**(4): 227–34.

Jacelon CS (2003) The dignity of elders in an acute care hospital. *Qualitative Health Research* **13**(4): 543–56.

Jacobson N (2007) Dignity and health: a review. *Social Science and Medicine* **64**(2): 292–302.

Jacobson N (2009) Dignity violation in healthcare. *Qualitative Health Research* **19**(11): 1536–47.

Lothian K, Philp I (2001) Maintaining the dignity and autonomy of older people in the healthcare setting. *BMJ* **322**(7287): 668–70.

Lundqvist A, Nilstun T (2007) Human dignity in paediatrics: the effects of healthcare. *Nursing Ethics* **14**(2): 216–28.

Matiti MR (2002) *Patient Dignity in Nursing: a phenomenological study*. Unpublished thesis. University of Huddersfield School of Education and Professional Development.

Matiti M, Sharman J (1999) Dignity: a study of pre-operative patients. *Nursing Standard* **14**(13–15): 32–5.

Matthews R, Callister LC (2004) Childbearing women's perceptions of nursing care that promotes dignity. *Journal of Obstetrics, Gynaecologic and Neonatal Nursing* **33**(4): 498–507.

Nordenfelt L (2003) Dignity of the elderly: an introduction. *Medicine, Healthcare and Philosophy* **6**(2): 99–101.

Öhlén J (2004) Violation of dignity in care-related situations. *Research and Theory for Nursing Practice* **18**(4): 371–85.

Patients Association (2009) *Patients . . . Not Numbers, People . . . Not Statistics*. London: Patients Association.

Picker Institute (2008) *The Challenge of Assessing Dignity in Care.* London: Help the Aged.

Pokorny ME (1989) *The Effect of Nursing Care on Human Dignity in the Critically Ill Adult.* Unpublished PhD thesis. University of Virginia.

Randers I, Mattiasson A (2004) Autonomy and integrity: upholding older adult patients' dignity. *Journal of Advanced Nursing* 45(1): 63–71.

Reed P (2007) *Dignity and the Child in Hospital.* Unpublished PhD thesis. University of Surrey.

Reed P, Smith P, Fletcher M, Bradding A (2003) Promoting the dignity of the child in hospital. *Nursing Ethics* 10(1): 67–76.

Royal College of Nursing (2008) *Defending Dignity: challenges and opportunities for nurses.* London: Royal College of Nursing.

Rylance G (1999) Privacy, dignity and confidentiality: interview study with structured questionnaire. *BMJ* 318(7179): 301.

Seedhouse D, Gallagher A (2002) Undignifying institutions. *Journal of Medical Ethics* 28: 368–72.

Sizmur S, Redding D (2009) *Core Domains for Measuring Inpatients' Experience of Care.* Oxford: Picker Institute Europe.

Slettebo A, Caspari S, Lohne V *et al* (2009) Dignity in the life of people with head injuries. *Journal of Advanced Nursing* 65(11): 2426–33.

Stabell A, Nåden D (2006) Patients' dignity in a rehabilitation ward: ethical challenges for nursing staff. *Nursing Ethics* 13(3): 236–48.

Stratton D, Tadd W (2005) Dignity and older people: the voice of society. *Quality in Ageing* 6(1): 37–45.

Street A (2001) Constructions of dignity in end-of-life care. *Journal of Palliative Care* 17(2): 93–101.

Turnock C, Kelleher M (2001) Maintaining patient dignity in intensive care settings. *Intensive and Critical Care Nursing* 17(3): 144–54.

Walsh K, Kowanko I (2002) Nurses' and patients' perceptions of dignity. *International Journal of Nursing Practice* 8(3): 143–51.

Watson J (1996) Watson's theory of transpersonal caring. In: Walker PH, Newman B (eds) *Blue Print for Use of Nursing Models – Education, Research, Practice and Administration.* New York: National League for Nursing Press, pp.141–84.

Webster C, Bryan K (2009) Older people's views of dignity and how it can be promoted in a hospital environment. *Journal of Clinical Nursing* 18(12): 1784–92.

Whitehead J, Wheeler H (2008) Patients' experience of privacy and dignity. Part 2: an empirical study. *British Journal of Nursing* 17(7): 457–64.

Widäng I, Fridlund B (2003) Self-respect, dignity and confidence: conceptions of integrity among male patients. *Journal of Advanced Nursing* 42(1): 47–56.

Widäng I, Fridlund B, Martenssen J (2008) Women patients' conceptions of integrity within healthcare: a phenomenographic study. *Journal of Advanced Nursing* 61(5): 540–8.

Woogara J (2004a) Patient' rights to privacy and dignity in the NHS. *Nursing Standard* 19(18): 33–7.

Woogara J (2004b) *Patient Privacy: an ethnographic study of privacy in NHS patient settings.* Unpublished PhD thesis. University of Surrey.

Index